His Change of Life

His Change of Life: Male Menopause and Healthy Aging with Testosterone

Chris D. Meletis, N.D. and Sara G. Wood, N.D.

Foreword by Jay H. Mead, M.D., FASCP

Complementary and Alternative Medicine

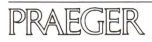

Westport, Connecticut
London

Library of Congress Cataloging-in-Publication Data

Meletis, Chris D.
   His change of life : male menopause and healthy aging with testosterone / Chris D. Meletis and Sara G. Wood; foreword by Jay H. Mead.
      p. ; cm.—(Complementary and alternative medicine, ISSN 1549-084X)
   Includes bibliographical references and index.
   ISBN 978–0–313–36023–7 (alk. paper)
   1. Climacteric, Male.   I. Wood, Sara, 1976–   II. Title.   III. Series: Complementary and alternative medicine (Westport, Conn.)
[DNLM: 1. Andropause—physiology.   2. Aging—physiology.   3. Hormone Replacement Therapy—adverse effects.   4. Naturopathy—methods.   5. Testosterone—secretion.   6. Testosterone—therapeutic use.   WJ 702 M519m   2009]
   RC884.M45   2009
   618.1′75—dc22   2008051893

British Library Cataloguing in Publication Data is available.

Library of Congress Catalog Card Number: 2008051893
ISBN: 978–0–313–36023–7
ISSN: 1549-084X

First published in 2009

Praeger Publishers, 88 Post Road West, Westport, CT 06881
An imprint of Greenwood Publishing Group, Inc.
www.praeger.com

Printed in the United States of America

∞™

The paper used in this book complies with the Permanent Paper Standard issued by the National Information Standards Organization (Z39.48–1984).

10 9 8 7 6 5 4 3 2 1

To the human body that is made of 50 to 100 trillion cells that work magnificently and tirelessly in unison to sustain our body and maintain overall peak performance. May each of our readers enjoy the Creative Power within their body, and choose to maximize its power and achieve their personal life goals.

Special acknowledgment to my wife and boys, you inspire me. To my parents: thanks for helping guide my path. To God, the creator of my mind, body, and spirit, thank you for the drive and passion to help others that you have instilled within my soul—it has allowed me to serve humanity. To all those that support DivineMedicine.com, my personal outreach to help improve the world's health one person at a time, thank you. To all my patients, you have blessed me with more knowledge and inspiration than all the book study that a physician can ever achieve. May we all be the masters of our bodies. If something doesn't feel right in your body, settle for nothing other than true and full wellness.—Chris D. Meletis, N.D.

To all the special men in my life, and especially my brother Grant, my father Cart, my Uncle Bruce, and Rob Ryan: I can't imagine life without any of you, **please** take care of yourselves. Thanks to my mom and my dad for always supporting me, even when my path was not the norm. Thank you to my patients for sharing their lives and their experiences, and making it all worthwhile. Thanks to Justin Sprung for contributing his artwork. And special thanks to Rob for putting up with the many late nights and still keeping the bed warm for me when I got home.—Sara G. Wood, N.D.

Contents

Foreword

If you have asked yourself, "Is my male vitality waning?"; or, if you find yourself paying more attention to the commercials that clutter the sports channels imploring us to be ready "when the time is right" and grab us with comments such as, "if you have an erection lasting four hours or longer go to the nearest emergency room," then Drs. Meletis and Wood wrote this book for you. It is a must read—it very well may save your life! "That is bold statement," you might say. I think not! The allopathic medical system is the third leading cause of death in the United States of America as reported in the *Journal of the American Medical Association* (JAMA 284:483–5). Of the 225,400 deaths in 2000 attributed to the medical system, 106,000 were caused by adverse drugs reactions. The pharmaceuticals hyped in those commercials can actually be deadly—read the package inserts. The approach back to wellness you will learn in this book uses safe natural therapies and non-synthetic hormones. Furthermore, you will learn that erectile dysfunction (ED), even though likely to be corrected with the therapies in this book, should be the least of your concerns. The metabolic consequences of andropause can be devastating.

As an allopathic physician who "jumped ship" over a decade ago and joined the fellowship of complementary practitioners, I am not only proud to have been asked to write this Foreword, I am excited to endorse this book and recommend it to my patients. The task Chris and Sara took upon themselves to write a comprehensive, yet understandable, book for the casual reader was indeed a challenge. The few books available on this subject, mainly written by well-meaning allopathic physicians, address, at best, only partial truths regarding andropause. Drs. Meletis and Wood lay out all of the truths based on current knowledge. They illuminate all of the facets of men's health issues. Their approach to treating andropause is absolutely comprehensive. It includes the use of human identical (bio-identical) hormones—testosterone you will likely recognize—and others critically important such as DHEA, progesterone and cortisol. The concept of hormone balancing is essential and key to their approach; also, the need for diagnostic testing and monitoring for therapeutic levels is emphasized. Not all diagnostic testing is "created equal." You will learn about saliva testing, the most accurate and yet the most often misunderstood of all testing modalities.

Their approach to wellness is holistic. If you have ever wondered about the influence of life style, nutrition, exercise, and herbal medicinal options in relation to declining hormones, these areas are superbly covered as well. These topics I read with great interest. My MD training did not include any substantive training in these areas. In fact, my allopathic medical education was essentially controlled by the pharmaceutical industry—Big Pharma. Not until I was exposed to Naturopathic Medicine, did I appreciate the limitation of my training. Naturopathic principles are now an integral part of my clinical practice because they are sound and effective. In fact, naturopathic medicine predates Big Pharma by decades.

Now, if you are wondering if this approach is safe, you can rest assured the authors adhere to the Hippocratic tenet: "Above all do no harm." Their intention is to repair your endocrine system (glands that produce all of your hormones) to its native function to the extent possible, and when complete repair is not in the cards, supplement it with bio-identical hormones to optimize physiology (the way we were meant to work) and no more. Achieving this natural balance will enhance your quality and quantity of life.

Do yourself, spouse, significant other, children or grandchildren a huge favor—read this book and join the thousands of males who daily enjoy the benefits of a more youthful vitality and the chance to add quality years to their lives.

Jay H. Mead, M.D., FASCP
Pathologist and Complementary Practitioner

Preface

All men may be created equal, give or take; but not all men feel equally well, healthy, or in control of their lives. Millions of men are not achieving their full life's potential due to diminishing health and countless medical conditions. An all-too-common theme for the slow and subtle loss of the male bravado, vim, and vigor is decreased testosterone levels and loss of function within the body. Before you reach over and dial the number on the screen for a "male enhancement" product, remember that you are not defined by one function, but rather the decreased ability to rise up to life's occasions is merely a sign of a bigger process going on in your body; a sign that you need to stand up and refuse to accept premature aging, to stop your life from slipping away.

This book is written to empower, encourage, and educate. Excellent health is readily achievable and our intention is to establish a platform from which **you** can take charge of **your life** and **your health.** We also want to remember (with reverence and respect) all the great guys who didn't have the knowledge or resources this book provides, and who faded into the sunset—tired, depressed, and prematurely aged—simply because they didn't know they had another option.

Let us remind you that though this book is written to empower you (and indeed we will certainly make many recommendations on how you can take control of your health) this information is not intended to be taken in lieu of seeing a doctor. The body is complex, and each and every one of us is different. You will be best served by sharing your knowledge with your doctor and allowing him or her to guide your care.

Introduction

As a general rule, women tend to be more proactive about their health, more willing to admit when they aren't feeling well, more aware of their symptoms, more informed about what is going on in their bodies, and more apt to seek medical care. And that's why this book isn't about, or for, women. We certainly don't discourage women from reading it, as the better they understand the male body the more they may be able to help and support the men in their lives: their brothers, fathers, grandfathers,

During my last year of medical school, I was working with a local doctor who treated a number of women for menopause. In fact, at the time, he had just finished a book on women's hormones. One of his long-standing patients finally managed to drag her husband in to see us and the first thing she reported was that he had "**lost his sparkle.**"

They had been married for many years, and had several children and grandchildren. He was recently retired, and was enjoying spending his time working in the garden and volunteering at church. Several of the grandchildren lived locally and he spent quite a bit of time with them. As we sat and listened, we slowly began to gather (from the wife, of course) the story of how this man had slipped from being a dynamic, energetic, productive father and grandfather to just going through the motions of life. He didn't report being unhappy, but his wife said that she never saw him smile anymore and even their 4-year-old granddaughter had asked about him.

Lo and behold, when his hormones were tested, he was low in testosterone!

husbands, and lovers. The symptoms of andropause (male menopause) affect men, but also have a dramatic effect on the people who love them. We have noticed that time after time, the men that do make it into our offices are primarily brought there by their wives and girlfriends. We have met men of all socioeconomic classes who are suffering, as andropause doesn't care what kind of car you drive or where you work. These men are Boy Scout leaders, bus drivers, powerful executives of large companies, involved members of the community, athletes, and fathers. These are capable men, providers for their families who take care of others, but who were neglecting their health, primarily because they just didn't know better. **This book is for those men**.

A good portion of this book will speak about testosterone and other hormones and their impact on all aspects of men's health. So let's start with the basics. A hormone is simply a chemical in the body that is secreted by one cell, and has an action on another cell. Unfortunately, many people associate the word hormone almost exclusively with women and such experiences as PMS, pregnancy, and menopause. Few people we talk to are aware that the hormone levels in men can change and fluctuate over time, and that they have some dramatic effects on their emotions, their body, and their mind. Though there is some literature out there about "male menopause" or "andropause," it's primarily found as a section of a larger article or book about menopause or hormones in general. Furthermore, this information is not usually found in mainstream sources; it's certainly not on ESPN. The bottom line is that most men out there are not exposed to vital information about their health. We wanted to create a book that is easy to read, easy to follow, and explains to the average guy about aging, hormones, and proactive health—and so here we are. During the writing process, the need for this information was confirmed time and time again as men and women who asked about the title or topic of the book became intrigued about the topic, bewildered that they hadn't heard about it before, and excited to learn more. It seems that the problem is even worse than we may have thought! **This book is for those people**.

A number of years ago, Garth Brooks sang a song about being "much too young to feel this damn old." Garth was less than 30 when he wrote that song, and yet it speaks to the essence of how men of all ages and all walks of life feel. There comes a time for most of us when we notice that activities that were once effortless require a little (or a lot) more work. Our bodies start to change, our memories slip, and we just don't have the stamina that we once did. We expect some of these things to occur as we age, but many men experience these changes years before their peers and decades before they expect. If this sounds familiar, then **this book is for you**!

Our goal here is to help you understand what is going on inside your body, and what you can do to look and feel your best for many years to come regardless of your age. We'll talk about metabolic pathways and specialized diagnostic tests, but we'll explain them so that you can use this information to communicate effectively with your physicians to ensure that you get the best care possible. We want to empower you so that you are aware of all of your resources and are educated about your body. We'll tell you stories of men just like you who discovered that their hormone levels had fallen far below optimal levels, how that made them feel, and what they did about it. Some of our stories are shared or collective experiences, although a few of them are unique to one of us and you'll notice we will switch to using the word "I" during those times. As you'll read in the book, much of the information that we'll present to you isn't new. Some of it will be new to **you,** but the research on men's hormones and their effects has been going on for decades. This comes as a surprise to many people who are just now hearing the word andropause or the concept of a "male menopause."

CHAPTER 1

Andropause: History, Incidence, and Effects

It is time to adopt a new perspective of what it means to be a healthy man in this new millennium. The concepts we are going to introduce are ones you will not likely hear from your average doctor. There is no question that this book will help change your life's trajectory and put you in charge of a large part of the "changes" in your life and your overall health and happiness.

Let's start with a phrase that most guys attribute to women: "the change of life." We've all heard this phrase used to describe the period of life when hormone levels begin to decline in WOMEN. This change of life has been documented by decades of research. It has been shown that there are VERY REAL physical and mental manifestations of depression, irritability, moodiness, and difficulty making decisions along with hot flashes, insomnia, and weight gain. So, big deal. The change of life merely describes menopause. Nope, think again. It's time for equality; these are the symptoms of "andropause." Yes, that is right, "male menopause." All of these symptoms occur with declining hormones in MEN as well as women! We've all seen hours and hours of sitcoms, movies, and daytime talk shows devoted to talking about menopause. You may not feel like you have very much in common with women in Oprah's audience discussing their water retention and hot flashes, but the truth is we all have more in common than we have recognized. In the past, when men in their forties or fifties experienced mood changes or depression, they were labeled as having a "Midlife Crisis," but isn't it plausible that men also have changes in hormone levels that affect their energy levels, their emotions, and their health? Just as women's ovaries stop producing hormones, the male testicles also go into hibernation, so to speak. They may not totally cease production, but they decrease their output significantly. In fact, all you have to do is look at the testosterone lab test reference ranges to see that the bar is set a lot lower for guys as they get older. The same exact numerical value may be below range for men until they reach a certain age when there is an adjustment in what is acceptable for a "normal" level of testosterone. "Normal" is not *optimal*. The divorce rate in this country is approaching 50 percent. That means it's likely that many of your friends or family members are divorced, and you may often find yourself in a group of people where everyone (or at least the majority of people) are divorced. By definition, *normal* means whatever is typical. Thus, this makes divorce normal. Of course, very few people would argue that divorce is optimal. Well, at least they wouldn't argue that before they get married!

We're not proposing that declining testosterone levels directly cause men to marry younger women or to suddenly purchase a convertible sports car, but the changing hormonal environment in their bodies can certainly account for changes in mood, vigor, and self-esteem. Just as a new Corvette won't solve these problems, neither will the little blue pills or other products that are advertised on late-night infomercials because the problem is bigger than that. For a woman, menopause can't be missed for it is marked by the end of her menstrual cycle. That makes it blatantly obvious that there are some big changes going on in her body, but maybe men aren't as different as we think! The definition of menopause is the date when one calendar year has passed since menstruation. Though this seems like an absolute date, even in a woman's body, hormones don't decline all of a sudden. Perimenopause is the time between when a woman first starts to notice changes or fluctuations in her cycle up until that first anniversary of her last period, and this process can last for several years. Perimenopause is often subtle, especially in the beginning. Surprise! The same thing is true for "male menopause"! The average guy doesn't just wake up one day and wonder where his muscle mass and bravado has gone, it just slowly slips away and, in fact, is an even slower process than for women!

It took years for the hormonal changes that occur in women throughout their lives to be studied and documented in medical research and literature. This fact should be very scary to any guy, because there are so many obvious hormonal "mile markers" for women: PMS, with its notable hormonal fluctuations; pregnancy, when hormones are turned upside down and it seems that the pregnant woman's emotions can turn on a dime; and, of course, the myriad symptoms that come with menopause. If you've ever lived with a woman who's pregnant, premenstrual, or menopausal, you can probably attest to the fact that you didn't need any scientific proof that something was going on in her body. The bottom line is that much has changed over the last few decades when it comes to gender equality, especially in the Western world. Equality is a two-way street, and this concept should certainly be extended to include healthcare.

When I (S. Wood) was first in medical school, there were a number of young doctors-to-be who were proclaiming that their interest was in "women's health." What they meant was that they were interested in treating primarily women, and treating them for conditions that were exclusively female: gynecological exams, breast health, and hormonal support. One first-year student in my class mentioned that he thought he was interested in going into "men's health." Hmmm, we all thought. That's unusual. What exactly does that mean? Well, he explained that he was interested in treating primarily men for conditions that were exclusive to men such as prostate health and issues relating to the penis and testicles. He was serious and is now practicing in California; and, true to his word, he is focusing on men. Of course, that makes growing his practice infinitely more difficult than the "women's health" doctors, as men don't go to the doctor nearly as often as women. In fact, *Angie's List*, a magazine that conducts surveys and publishes lists of popular and reputable service providers including medical professionals, recently did a survey and found that 25 percent of the men that responded avoided going to the doctor.[1] We'd like to see this movement for equality spread to include more complete healthcare for men. At the turn of the century, women were only expected to outlive men by one year or so. They are now expected to outlive men by approximately five years! We now see women in regions of the world where there is combat, women in top executive business positions, and it even seems inevitable that we will have a woman in the White House within the next few years, as both parties have viable female candidates. So, isn't it about time that that our hormones are all treated equally?

> There are many names for the pattern of declining hormones seen in men as they age:
>
> - Hypogonadism
> - Climacteric
> - Somatopause
> - Viropause—decline in virility
> - ADAM—androgen deficiency in aging men
> - PADAM—partial androgen deficiency in aging men
> - Male menopause
> - Andropause
> - Late onset hypogonadism

The truth of the matter is that total testosterone levels decline in men at the rate of approximately 1.6 percent per year starting at age 30.[2] Yes, 30. And that's just the rate that they fall without additional influences, but we all know that we don't live in a vacuum. There are innumerable situations that exacerbate this situation. You may be wondering why you haven't heard about this before. You may be asking yourself why somebody didn't tell you that you had hormones, too! Well, we're here to explain how these fluctuations in hormone levels are affecting you and the men you know, and what you can do about it.

It seems that there has been great debate about naming the phenomenon of declining hormone levels in men. Decrease in the function of the gonads (testes or ovaries) and, therefore, a decrease in the hormones that they produce is broadly called hypogonadism. This occurs at many stages of development for many different reasons. Hypogonadism that is caused by aging is the specific condition that we are referencing, and has been given many different names though the years. The symptoms of andropause were first described as "climacteric disease in males" by H. Halford in 1813 and reintroduced into modern medical terminology in the 1930s by A. A. Werner. In the late 1930s, subsequent to the isolation of various androgens, reports were published on the treatment of the male climacteric and its accompanying melancholic symptoms with **testosterone.**[3] In 1944, Heller and Myers again described "the male climacteric" in the *Journal of the American Medical Association.*[4] Climacteric is defined as "a period of decrease of reproductive capacity in men and women, culminating, in women, in the menopause."[5] Climacteric is also used to describe the period of maximum ripening in fruit, the final physiological process that marks the end of fruit maturation before the process of decomposition begins. Now we don't know any men that appreciate the idea that they are on the downslide or the fast track to old age and infirmity, nor should they. This may have been a more valid likeness when this particular paper was written in the 1940s.[6] Back then, the life expectancy in the United States was only 62, but today the average life expectancy of a man is 75 and can be even higher if you take care of yourself and have a little luck from genetics. There are currently almost 5 million Americans over the age of 85, and that doesn't include any of the "baby boomers" who will likely make this number jump significantly in 20 years. Of course, who wants to stop at 85? There are currently more than 84,000 people in the United States who are at least 100 years old! We mention genetics, and though the inherited traits you receive from your family are important, it's also important to remember that genetics may load the gun, but diet and lifestyle pull the trigger. Or put another way, you might have a family history of heart disease, but that does not mean you have to accept that history as your own, unless you don't do anything about it. After all, **inaction is the active process of doing nothing.** Don't sit back and let yourself become prematurely old, depressed, or sick. The decline of hormones certainly does not need to result in you feeling like your life is winding down. In fact, this phase of life, when many of the daily stresses of raising children and working for a living are in the past, can be the most rewarding for many people.

Symptoms of testosterone deficiency include:

- Fatigue
- Depression
- Anxiety
- Decreased libido
- Erectile dysfunction
- Night sweats
- Sleep disturbances
- Heart disease
- Metabolic syndrome
- Breast enlargement
- Thinning hair
- Elevated triglycerides
- Decreased mental sharpness
- Loss of muscle tone
- Abdominal weight gain
- Decreased urinary flow
- Forgetfulness
- Osteopenia (weakening bones)
- Mild anemia
- Diabetes

"Male menopause" doesn't seem a very fitting name since menopause, when we break it down, is a direct reference to the end of menses, as "meno" comes from the Greek *mens* meaning monthy and "pause" from the Greek *pausis* meaning cessation. Plus, men deserve their own name, not just to name their condition after their female counterparts! "Andropause" is a commonly used term, and since "andro" means male or masculine, andropause literally means a suspension of maleness. Since the purposes that testosterone serves in the body are often those qualities that we most strongly associate with masculinity—hair growth, sexual appetite, acquisition of muscle mass, drive and zeal for life, the proverbial "eye of the tiger" as well as less desirable qualities such as aggression—a decrease in these hormones (and subsequently a decrease in the "male" traits) does more or less equate to a decrease in masculinity. Now we see why this can drive a man to start skydiving or invest in a race car—no man wants to feel or be viewed as though he is losing his masculinity! So, what is actually happening in the body during this time we call andropause? As we age, hormone levels decline, but this occurs differently in men than women. For women, estrogen and progesterone levels decline relatively quickly during her perimenopausal years. They stay at a relatively constant level from puberty throughout her life until dropping sometime in her forties or fifties. In contrast, testosterone levels in men begin disappearing much earlier and the loss is a gradual process. You can think of it like this: a pinhole leak in your gas tank will eventually leave you stranded on the side of the road just as a dime-sized hole will. You may make it a few more miles, but the end result is the same.

Testosterone is the main androgen or "male sex hormone" found in the human body. Both men and women have testosterone, just as both sexes have estrogen and progesterone or the "female sex hormones," but men have a greater ratio of testosterone to the others. In fact, speaking of equality, to be fair we wanted to share with you that testosterone helps women with many of the same things that it helps men with. We often have women in their 30s and 40s who come into our practice and are working hard to be fit, exercising aggressively, working with personal trainers, and really watching their diets, but still aren't getting the results they feel they should be getting. Or sometimes they come into the office because they just aren't "in the mood" as often as they used to be. A large percentage of these women turn out to be deficient in testosterone when tested. Don't get the wrong idea: we aren't helping anyone "juice" or increase their testosterone levels to super-physiological levels, but a little adjustment can make a huge difference. There are many hormones that play a part for both genders, and we'll cover that in later chapters, but for now let's just talk a little about men and testosterone to make it simple.

The gradual hormone decline starts as early as age 30, and, after that, testosterone levels in men drop by more than 1 percent per year, leaving a man in his seventies with half the testosterone he had when he was 25. Many of these men are not yet experiencing the symptoms associated with this drop, but by the time they reach 50, they are noticing a lack of energy, loss of libido, impaired memory, depression, erectile dysfunction, and many other symptoms. The decrease in testosterone level is coupled with an increase in sex hormone binding globulin (SHBG), a protein that binds to testosterone (and other hormones), leaving an even smaller amount of the hormone free (or unbound) in circulation. It is this free testosterone that is biologically active, or available to the target tissues. But wait, there's more: many disease processes, injuries, lifestyle choices, and environmental factors adversely affect these levels so that they can fall even lower. Do you know any 30- to 40-something-year-old men with high stress levels who don't get enough exercise and eat out too often? Maybe some of them drink more often than they should or smoke? Of course you do. If you don't find that guy in the mirror, then you almost certainly have a brother or a neighbor or a college buddy who meets most of those criteria. And how often do men this age go to the doctor? You know as well as we do that the answer is not very often. You can see how we create a cycle where our lifestyle is often detrimental to our hormone levels, and, in turn, our declining hormone levels are detrimental to our health. We're not asserting that the only reason it's not healthy to smoke like the Marlboro Man and enjoy a fourth meal every night is because of the effects it has on hormone levels. There are many ways that these behaviors can affect our health, and impacting hormone levels is just one of them. Furthermore, external factors such as hormones found in our food, or hormone disruptors that come from pesticides and preservatives, are major contributors to altered hormone levels. These aggravating influences may explain why many indigenous cultures around the world don't seem to suffer from the same symptoms of andropause and menopause that we do in western society. So it's not just age that is working against us—there are a lot of factors affecting our hormone levels that we **can** control.

Speaking of age, we all know that there is no way to avoid the passing of years. Though time travel makes for an interesting book, movie, or TV series, the reality is that we can't stop time. What we can do is change what those years do to our bodies, and how we look and feel at any given age. Not all 60-year-olds are created equal. A friend was just telling me the other day of a neighbor whom she recently discovered is only 56 years old. She had assumed he was in his seventies due to his declining health and vitality. On the flip side, I (S. Wood) have a patient whom I would have pinned to be in her fifties, only to find out that she just turned 70! I'm sure we all have examples of both of these extremes. It's not just physical health that is indicative of someone's age, there's also the young attitude that many people are able to maintain well into their elder years. Barbara Walters did a special television show on aging.[7] During the show, she interviewed a number of people who were over the age of 100 and found that one thing that they had in common was a positive attitude and optimistic outlook on life. They had suffered from many of the same ailments that had taken the lives of their friends and family members. There were cancer survivors and heart transplant patients and diabetics. The difference was their approach to the problems they faced. Our point here is that age really is just a number and there are vast differences between chronological age and biological age. We are living longer than we ever have in the past. Former generations died of infectious diseases that we rarely even hear of, let alone consider a threat anymore. One hundred years ago, most Americans lived to be an average of 47 years old. We now live to be in our mid-to-late seventies, so we are all living many years beyond when our hormones begin to decline. Why does this matter? We have extended our lives through technology, industry, and medical

There is a BIG difference between chronological age, the age on your driver's license, and biological age, the actual wear and tear that has occurred to the 75 trillion cells that make up your body. With just a little inclination, you can change your biological age by staying more active physically and mentally.

research, but by failing to address our hormonal health we are literally extending the last years of our lives, instead of the vibrant middle years.

The chronic diseases that we suffer from result in compromised hormone levels that affect our physical health as well as our mental and emotional well-being, rendering it more and more difficult to maintain an optimistic, fun outlook on life. There is no reason for a decrease in masculinity as men age. Aging is, of course, the process of getting older, and no, there is nothing we can do about it. That means 40 will always be 40 and 65 always 65, but there is no reason that we have to let the number of years we have been alive define the way we feel, the things we do, and our quality of life. Now, you may be thinking of those pictures you see of octogenarians in bodybuilding poses with more muscles than a college athlete. If this is what you are after, you can probably find a doctor out there who can help you with it, but there's a whole world between the muscle-bound super grandpa and a man who's limping around on a cane and looks as though he might blow over if a bus comes by too fast.

Monitoring and maintaining normal hormone levels is as important to your health as it is to your wife, girlfriend, or sister. How do you go about pursuing this avenue? How do you know what your hormone levels are, and what can you do about it? These are all questions that this book is intended to help you with. Of course, you will need the assistance of your primary care physician; he or she can help by ordering the tests you need from your local lab. There are several ways to test hormones; it can be done in urine, in serum, or in saliva. If your doctor isn't familiar with these tests or doesn't want to order them for you, you can order them yourself. Think of it this way: are you worth a couple of hundred dollars? Of course you are! You'd spend that money on a golf trip or basketball tickets or cable TV without batting an eye. You spend money to have fun, right? Well, you'll have more fun if you are in optimal shape. This is literally a discovery that can change the way you feel and live for the rest of your life! You can get the testing done, get the evidence and proof, and then share them with your doctor. You shouldn't let anyone stop you from knowing what your hormone levels are, now that you know to test them! We will go into these various methods in more detail and what their individual advantages are. We will also tell you about other

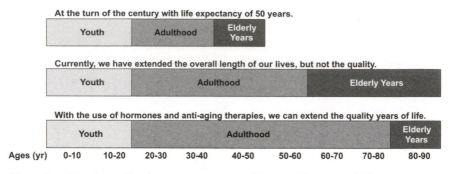

Figure 1.1 Supplementing hormones can extend the quality years of life.

tests you should monitor such as the prostate-specific antigen (PSA) to check the health of your prostate and cardiac markers to keep an eye on your heart function. In addition to deciding what the best method of testing may be for you, the time of day that you give a sample may be important. Testosterone levels (along with many other hormone levels) have a natural circadian rhythm, meaning that the levels fluctuate throughout the day. Lab tests are like taking a snapshot of what is going on in the body at the exact time that the sample is given. Testosterone levels are highest in the morning, so that's the best time to take the "snapshot." If you know what your levels are at their highest, you know what the best case scenario is.

So, what can you do about it if your levels are low? There are many different approaches, although the first that comes to mind for most people is hormone treatment with an injection, an oral testosterone compound, a lozenge, or a transdermal testosterone gel, cream, or patch. Not all testosterone is created equal. Time has proven that there is a very significant difference in the way the body responds to synthetic hormones as opposed to bio-identical hormones. Testosterone (bio-identical or otherwise) requires a prescription and should always be monitored by a physician.

> Bio-identical hormones are made by compounding pharmacies and are identical in structure to the hormones that our body produces from cholesterol. There will be more detail on this in later chapters when we get to discussing what you can do about your declining hormone levels.

Of course, many people are afraid of testosterone supplementation, associating it with increased aggressiveness or other behaviors exhibited by anabolic steroid users. The truth is that it is very safe to supplement testosterone to achieve optimal **physiologic** levels under a doctor's care, but this isn't the only answer. "Physiologic" refers to the amount of a substance that is normally found in the body, meaning that it is not higher than you are capable of producing on your own under optimal conditions. Sometimes changing diet and lifestyle habits alone can have a significant impact on hormones and may be a good place to start, especially if you are young. Herbs and dietary supplements can play a large role, as we'll cover in chapter 9. Keep in mind that there is no such thing as a panacea, and even testosterone supplementation can have some negative effects, especially if too much is taken. The goal is to get your levels back into the upper middle of the "normal" range and level the playing field with the guys you may hoop, golf, or play tennis with, or even those guys you are competing with at work. As with all things, moderation is the key. There are some dangers to testosterone supplementation; testosterone can significantly decreases sperm production, for example, and can temporarily render you infertile and cause your testicles to shrink in size. These symptoms will generally be reversed if you stop supplementing, but they are certainly something to be aware of, and of course to discuss with your wife or girlfriend. If you are still thinking of having children, testosterone replacement may not be for you, although there are a number of herbs and nutritional supplements and other compounds that can enhance endogenous (meaning it comes from you) testosterone production and not adversely affect fertility. Other herbs limit the conversion of testosterone to estrogen, which is one of the things that happens as we get older and is one of the many mechanisms behind the symptoms and problems associated with changes in hormone levels. But we're going to get to all of that soon.

Remember the old adage "an ounce of prevention is worth a pound of cure"? You don't have to wait until you are suffering along with the other tens of thousands of men with low hormone levels. There are many things you can do to ensure that you maintain optimal hormone levels well into your later years. The earlier you are starting, the better! Don't put this book down and wait for problems to arise—be proactive and on top of your health. You'll save yourself a lot of effort, time, pain, and money! It's easy to feel invincible when you are young and in your prime, but just as it's a good idea to start a savings account to provide you with income as you age and retire, you should put the same amount of effort and care into your health, and maintaining healthy hormone levels is a great place to start. Have you ever thought of aging as a disease? This may be a new concept to you, but just give it a chance. Cutting-edge physicians around the world are literally treating the disease of aging. We're not talking about some science fiction story where we suspend aging and live forever, but rather slowing the physiological processes that result in the symptoms that we commonly attribute to "getting old." So, read on if you are experiencing some of the symptoms we have listed and want to know what you can do about it; read on if you are curious about what your hormones are doing, or **not** doing in your body; and read on if you want to do what you can to age with style and grace, energy and vitality.

> If your thumb was throbbing with pain and you asked three friends what to do for it, one might say take Advil and another might say take Tylenol, but the wisest friend will tell you to remove the splinter that was causing the pain to start with.

"Tim" is a 48-year-old man who began to notice a decline in his energy a couple of years ago. He was tested at that time and treated for a thyroid deficiency. Recently, Tim felt as though the same symptoms were reappearing and inquired about adjusting his dose of thyroid hormone. His labs indicated that his thyroid levels were adequate, which prompted a few more questions. Literally, the first few things he said as he sat down in the chair were "my brain feels like it's stuck in molasses and last Saturday I literally cried for much of the day and I'm not sure why." When asked about his libido, he reported he "couldn't care less." When told about the other hormones he had (in addition to thyroid) and asked if he had ever had these levels checked, he seemed to get excited. No one had ever told him that he could be suffering from a changing hormonal environment much like the women his age; yet, he was experiencing several of the most common and obvious symptoms of andropause! A quick saliva test revealed that his testosterone levels were significantly below where they should be and his estrogen levels were rising!

Imagine how much more you could get done, how much smoother your life would run if you could think as clearly as you did when you were in college (and I'm not talking about the mornings after those keg parties). Picture how a boost to your sex drive and your—ahem—performance capabilities could give your relationship a little shot of energy. Envision how much easier it would be to get the yard work done, or play with the kids on the weekends if you weren't so fatigued. These scenarios are all real and attainable. The "Tim" is a real guy (though that's not his real name), and you'll meet many other men in this book that will likely sound familiar. We don't want to sound like an infomercial you find on TV in the middle of the night where they go on and on about how great some miracle product is. We're not selling you any miracle product, but simply want to introduce you to the idea that your hormones are affecting your body, your mind, and your emotions every day and you don't have to just sit back and get **old**—you can take the bull by the horns and just get **older**.

NOTES

1. "Going to the Doctor: Men vs. Women, 10 TV News," Tuesday, September 2, 2008, http://www.10tv.com/live/content/homegarden/stories/2008/09/02/angieslist_doctor.html?sid=102.

2. Feldman, H.A., C. Longcope, C.A. Derby, et al., "Age trends in the level of serum testosterone and other hormones in middle-aged men: Longitudinal results from the Massachusetts male aging study," *J Clin Endocrinol Metab* (2002): 87: 589–598.

3. Altschule, M.D., and K.J. Tillotson, "The use of testosterone in the treatment of depression," *N Engl J Med* (1948): 239:1036–1038. Lamar, C.P, "Clinical endrocrinology

of the male: with special reference to the male climacteric," *J Fla Med Assoc* (1940): 26:398–404.

4. Heller, C.G., G.B. Myers, "The Male climacteric: Its symptomatology, diagnosis and treatment," *JAMA* (1944): 126:472–77.

5. http://www.dictionary.com.

6. http://www.census.gov/Press-Release/www/releases/archives/facts_for_features_special_editions/004210.html.

7. *Live to 150, Can You Do It? Secrets to Living Longer with Barbara Walters*, ABC News, April 1, 2008, http://abcnews.go.com/health/longevity/story?id=4544003&page=1.

CHAPTER 2

The Controversy: Myth or Malady?

Andropause. Male menopause. Viropause. The male climacteric. It doesn't matter what you call it, the facts are that testosterone and other androgen hormone levels decline as men age, leading to overt signs and symptoms of infirmity. Though to many of you this book may be the first you have heard of this phenomenon, it's important to remember that until relatively recently we didn't see such a dramatic effect on men's lives...because many didn't live long enough to experience it. Remember, just 100 years ago the life expectancy for men was less than 50. Furthermore, it's important to remember that, generally speaking, men are MUCH less likely than women to go to the doctor for complaints such as fatigue or loss of libido. In part, this is because many believe fatigue is just part of life, and most men don't readily discuss the topic of libido. Many of the signs and symptoms of the climacteric process are very similar between men and women: they both experience an increase in body fat, a decrease in their libido and sense of well being, and an increase in incidence of cardiovascular disease, osteoporosis, and prostate or breast cancer. For men, the changing hormones result in a decrease in testosterone and a subsequent increase in estrogen, while in women the exact opposite occurs: their estrogen levels decline while their testosterone levels often rise! So what makes this process more "real" for women? The simple answer is NOTHING. There are measurable biochemical changes going on in the bodies of women AND men.

Well then, why is there so much controversy over whether or not this condition really exists? With a woman, there is the dramatic cessation of menses that makes it blatantly obvious that changes are occurring in her body. This has been known since the beginning of human existence, and though there have historically been many different cultural ideas of what was occurring, or what it meant, it was undeniable that something was different. With men, the changes aren't as

The **Quest Diagnostics Labs** reference range for free testosterone in serum (blood levels) in men ages 18–69 is 46 to 224 ng/dL, while the reference range for women of the same age group is 0.2 to 5.0 ng/dL.

Labrix Clinical Services states the reference range for testosterone in saliva as 30.1 to 142.5 pg/ml for men and 6.0–49 pg/ml for women. How do you measure up? You may not be below this range, but imagine how different you would feel if you were in the upper half of the range instead of at the bottom end. You aren't looking to have the hormone levels of an 18-year-old again, but making sure your hormone levels aren't scraping the bottom or even lower is a good idea. Checking to see that all of your testosterone isn't being converted into estrogen or bound up by SHBG is worthwhile as well! Remember, you don't have to be in your late forties or early fifites to start suffering the consequences of andropause. In clinical practice we routinely see guys that are in the early to mid-thirties beginning to manifest symptoms.

-www.questdiagnostics.com
-www.labrix.com

obvious to start with until one day, typically years after the time testosterone levels started dropping, a guy looks in a mirror and says to himself, "How in the world has this happened?" There is no single symptom that is the hallmark of the aging process for men. As mentioned before, the decline in hormones for men is often a very gradual process that makes it more difficult to see what is happening when compared to the more rapid drop that occurs in women. Have you ever heard the boiling frog theory? Studies that began in the 1880s found that if you put a frog in cold water and raise the temperature very gradually, that you can actually boil the frog alive. It won't jump out because it doesn't detect danger that is so gradual. On the other hand, if you put a live frog directly into hot water, it will jump out because it perceives the danger. Because women's hormones typically change more quickly, they notice a dramatic difference, even before they stop having a period.

Andropause	Menopause
↓ Testosterone	↓ Estrogen
↑ Body Fat	
↓ Sense of Well Being	
↑ Cardiovascular Disease	
↑ Prostate Cancer	↑ Breast Cancer
↑ Osteoporosis	
↓ Libido	

Figure 2.1 Men and women experience many of the same symptoms as their hormone levels change.

Men, on the other hand, have such a gradual change in testosterone levels (remember it's just over 1 percent per year) that they adapt to the changes and often don't even notice that they don't feel as well as they should. While many of the indications of andropause are similar to menopause (such as fatigue, hot flashes, and mood swings), the mere absence of a symptom that is unique to the condition makes it harder to define. What we're saying is that both sexes experience a wide range of symptoms that could be attributed to a number of causes. Take for example decreased mental clarity. Stress, nerve damage, atherosclerosis, infection, lack of sleep, side effects of medications, liver toxicity, and, of course, hormonal imbalance can all be possible underlying reasons that someone could be experiencing a "foggy brain." So when someone has a general feeling like this, they may attribute it to a number of causative factors. Conversely, there is really only one common explanation for why middle-aged women stop having a monthly period. It's like a big red flag (pardon the pun). There is no mystery as to what is going on: the alterations in monthly cycle often point in the direction of hormones as a cause of many of the additional problems that a woman may be having during that time. There is no "call sign" for men, no single symptom that stands out above the rest as uniquely due to declining hormones, so it's a much harder puzzle to decipher. The symptoms of andropause aren't as obvious, and, until relatively, recently symptoms have been all we had to go on. It has only been the last 50 years or so that we have had the ability to test for testosterone and other hormone levels in the body. Laboratory testing for testosterone became widely available after World War II, but even

---

"Dan" came in complaining of severe depression, fatigue, and insomnia. During the initial interview, he further disclosed that he had been prescribed Zetia for hyperlipidemia from his cardiologist and Prozac for depression. Upon further inquiry, he revealed casually that "oh, by the way" he also had "no sex drive." He had been seeing several doctors for his assortment of ailments, but no one had offered to check his hormone status.

His exhaustive lab testing uncovered a free testosterone level that was only 50 percent of "normal" as well as low cortisol levels and low thyroid.

Dan was treated with topical bio-identical testosterone and progesterone cream twice daily, DHEA orally, and pregnenolone, arginine, and thyroid hormone as well as advised to do squats and straight leg raises to build muscle.

In the first month, he noticed an improvement in all of his complaints by more than 25 percent and has continued to improve with each subsequent follow-up visit.

Contributed by Gerald W. Miller, MD, a board-certified, anti-aging physician and integrative physician specializing in nutrition and dietary counseling therapeutics in Beaverton, OR.

though we had developed the technology to test for the hormone, the test isn't employed very often. Many men who are experiencing the symptoms associated with low testosterone simply chalk it up to aging or being out of shape and never even see a doctor for it, and far too many doctors simply prescribe the latest pharmaceutical that has been developed for the symptom without looking into what may be causing the problem in the first place.

In 2006, the Mulligan study measured the testosterone levels of 2,162 men over the age of 45 who were already going in to their primary care physicians for another reason. They found that 836 of these men, almost 39 percent, had low testosterone levels.[1] That means that more than one-third of men who are seeing their doctor for cardiovascular problems, respiratory issues, diabetes, high cholesterol, high blood pressure or other complaints **also** had low testosterone levels. This study raises the question of whether or not testosterone levels should be done as a screening tool in men of that age group. Another study done in Boston, Massachusetts, on randomly chosen men between the ages of 30 and 70 found that 1 in 20 of 1,486 men surveyed and tested had measured low testosterone levels **coupled with symptoms** associated with andropause and a vast majority of these men (about 88 percent) were not receiving treatment.[2] The most important point of this study is that at least 1 in 4 guys over the age of 30 have measurably low levels of testosterone even if they aren't feeling it yet. Another paper from the same study found that while age increased the likelihood of low testosterone, waist circumference had a strong inverse relationship to measured testosterone levels[3]: the higher the waist circumference, the lower the testosterone levels. If fatigue, depression, decreased libido, heart disease, metabolic syndrome, or diabetes are creeping into your life or the lives of your friends or family members, it's time to look a little deeper at the cause. DO NOT ACCEPT "oh, I am just getting older." It is time to level the playing field and bring you or your friend back to "manufacturing specifications." After all, it is only fair that men should have the same advantage of hormone balancing and understanding about their hormones that women do! Maintaining normal physiologic levels of testosterone and other hormones can help ward off a myriad of unnecessary affliction and diseases. **THIS IS A REAL CONDITION!** Real suffering. Real disease. Real risk. You may not be experiencing very many of the effects of andropause yet, but don't wait until these symptoms are weighing you down. **Be proactive** and get your testosterone levels measured. It is good for your heart, muscles, waistline, and, of course, your sex life. You are already on the right track just by reading this book. In just the few short hours it will take you to flip through these pages you will empower yourself with knowledge that will change your life and the lives of many of your friends and family. If your doctor does not want to measure your levels, take charge and get the levels measured yourself. See our resource section at the back of the book.

Another argument that people often use when disputing the existence of andropause is that many men have proven to be fertile late into their lives. There are reports of modern men fathering children into their nineties, and Abraham was said to be 127 when his wife Sarah died and yet he still fathered six children with his third wife![4] These stories lead many people to the conclusion that everything must be fine if those little sperm are still swimming! Fertility is not equal to virility, and just because it is theoretically possible for men to father children so late in their lives doesn't mean that it occurs very often. Of course just to be fair, with the exception of Hugh Hefner and a man in India who had his twenty-first child last year at the age of 90, most men that age aren't given the opportunity to test their sperm count as men in their sixties, seventies, eighties, and beyond are usually sleeping with women close to their own age who are no longer fertile. The fact of the matter is that sperm count does decline with age, making the likelihood of conception more and more difficult, yet not completely impossible. Infertility is on the rise in general, and one-fourth to one-third of couples experiencing fertility problems find that the origin of the problem is the male partner. Though fertility and virility are often

Would you believe that the effects of testosterone are so far-reaching that fluctuating levels can even affect the stock market? Yep, we said the stock market. Dr. Rob Stein, from the University of Cambridge, did a study following testosterone levels and stock market traders in London. It seems that their morning testosterone levels were increased on days when they made particularly profitable trades. His theory is that when the trader's testosterone levels are high, it makes them more likely to take profitable risks. The same study also found that the trader's cortisol levels (a stress hormone) rose with volatility in the market or with their individual trading results. There are few jobs out there with as much stress as an on-the-floor market trader, and the rising cortisol levels are indicative of the stress level. The point is, the cortisol numbers are reflecting the stress we expect that they are under, but the testosterone levels are measured **before** the successful trades on the market, indicating that it is the hormone levels affecting behavior, not the other way around.

Source: J.M. Coates, J. Herbert Endogenous, "Steroids and financial risk taking on a London trading floor," PNAS 2008 105: 6167–6172.

used synonymously, there is a difference. Virility is your manhood, like a measure of your machismo, your proverbial "get up and go." This word describes something more than simply the ability to procreate; it's that essence of men. Virility smells like Old Spice, looks like John Wayne, and sounds like Sam Elliott. Regardless of what you look like, how you dress, or your individual scent, you've got some of it. Fertility is a much clearer concept. Either you are fertile and can father a child, or you aren't. Some men aren't very virile, yet are still fertile; and other men may not be fertile, but maintain their virility. In a very basic sense, testosterone is what makes up your virility, whereas sperm count is responsible for your fertility. Yes, we know that we are over-simplifying things a little bit, but have some patience. This is only chapter 2; we have a lot more material to cover!

We've mentioned it a couple of times, but just to reiterate in case you were dozing off, the age that testosterone levels begin to decline is 30. This means that at an age when many men are still playing video games, living in a bachelor pad, and just beginning to entertain thoughts of settling down, their hormone levels are already starting to fall. By the time men are in their mid-to-late forties, at a time when they are struggling with raising teenagers or dealing with aging parents and need all the energy they can muster, they are likely experiencing the fatigue and declining health that is associated with waning hormones. For men in their sixties, a time when the kids are likely out of the house, and they should be taking advantage of alone time with their loved one, the decreased libido, depression, and erectile dysfunction prevent them from fully appreciating the "golden years" that they worked so many years to arrive at with grand anticipation.

If hormones begin to decline at such an early age, leaving what can be several decades with low hormone levels, should we do anything about it or chalk it up to just a normal aging process? Is aging a natural process through which we should pass gracefully and not interfere? Or is aging a result of the pathological breakdown of physiological processes that we should control to the best of our ability? Why not? Medical intervention has lengthened our lives, so shouldn't we use it to increase the quality of life, especially in those later years? Who wants to live to be 100 or 110 years old if the last twenty to thirty years are spent in a nursing home unable to walk, think clearly, or use the toilet without assistance! Seriously, that's not what we strive for when we say we want to live long lives. Contrary to most of the American healthcare system that focuses on disease management, much of our practices focus on wellness and healthy aging. Wouldn't you rather focus on actual prevention and building the body strong from the cellular level than wait until you are in a disease state and have to recover? Waiting until you are sick to start working on your health is like playing your third-string players in a football game for the first half and then putting your starters in after halftime when you are two touchdowns in the hole. If you work hard enough, chances are you can still recover and win the game, but it's a much harder struggle. Wouldn't it make more sense to play your best guys from the beginning of the game? Modern medicine and community health has provided us with the ability to avoid fatal infections, reduce the daily dangers that we encounter, and even repair or replace organs that have been damaged or worn out. Just a few generations ago, people died of infections such as polio and malaria, and a few generations before that people were killed by wild animals and exposure to the elements. These days we live longer, but die from chronic disease and the effects that those years take on our bodies. The missing link in modern healthcare has been not looking far enough into the future.

> "Forty is the old age of youth, fifty is the youth of old age." —Victor Hugo

As mentioned, we have drugs and surgeries to save or to sustain a life, yet as we all see by looking around us, nothing has been put in place to **prevent** us from getting fat, slow, arthritic, and depressed; the pivotal word here is *prevent*. It is far better to avoid running over a nail than to keep patching the tire. Let's work on maintaining energy, vitality, and strength throughout our lives. We're not talking about making people look like they are 20 for eternity. From Botox® to tummy tucks, nose jobs to breast augmentation, Americans spent $13.2 billion on cosmetic procedures in 2007 alone![5] But changing the way you look is not likely to change the way you feel long term, and it certainly isn't going to change your risk for disease. There is nothing wrong with aging, and no reason why people shouldn't be proud of their age. In most cultures, aging is rewarded with respect from the community because with age comes wisdom, patience, and insight that, let's face it, we just don't have when we're younger. There are many advantages to aging. For many people, this means retirement, more time with their loved ones, or time spent doing what they love. This may

> "It's not about how long you live, but how you live long." —Michael Klentze, MD

mean weekends with your grandkids or a week alone fly-fishing in some river. The point here is that we aren't advocating the use of hormones to create an artificial environment in your body, but paying attention to your hormonal health can help you feel better, prevent disease, live longer, and as a bonus side effect, generally look better.

Have you ever given much thought to aging? Chances are it's crossed your mind a time or two regardless of your age. Maybe it's been as simple as finding yourself with some new lower back pain after doing an activity you once thought of as routine, or noticing that neither you nor your friends move as quickly or are as agile as you once were. Remember when a pickup game of basketball was no big deal or raking the lawn was something you did quickly before moving onto the rest of your day instead of becoming your primary Saturday activity? Maybe you've suffered from some significant health problems, experienced a heart attack, or been told you have high blood pressure and you thought, "Here it is, I'm getting old." Age is often one of those processes we just accept as fact and dismiss, kind of like gravity. Just as we can count on gravity holding us to the ground every morning when we roll out of bed, we can count on aging slowing

biological age -
n, the age determined by physiology rather than chronology. Factors include changes in the physical structure of the body as well as changes in the performance of motor skills and sensory awareness.

chronologic age -
n, age determined by the passage of time since birth.

us down, clogging our arteries, and eventually taking our lives, right? Wrong! You don't have to accept this as an absolute truth. What exactly causes aging, and what can we do about it? Now keep in mind that when we refer to aging, we're referring to biological age. Chronological age is the literal number of years, months, days, and minutes you have been alive. Obviously, there is nothing you can do about your chronological age short of lying to the DMV about your birthday, and what good is that going to do? Biological age is a number determined by your **physiology** rather than **chronology**; it is a rough estimate of how old most people would be in the same physical shape and can give us a much better idea of how long a person is likely to live than simply the date on his or her birth certificate. You can enjoy a youthful biological age that is significantly less than your chronological age if you tend to your health. Likewise, you can suffer from premature and accelerated aging that makes you look and feel much older than you may be chronologically. There are many theories on aging that we will explore in a few chapters and most of them are not mutually exclusive, meaning that these processes are likely to all be occurring simultaneously, resulting in the net effect we define as aging. So, when asked if andropause is a real condition or simply a symptom of getting older and is there anything we can do about it, the answer is yes, yes, and yes. Yes, andropause is a symptom of getting older. Yes, it is a real condition. And YES, there is a lot that we can do.

Andropause Assessment

Give yourself a score for each of the following symptoms: 0 - not a problem; 1 - occurs occasionally; 2 - happens frequently, causes a problem in my life; 3 - severe, debilitating.

Have you been experiencing the following:

1. Low energy or fatigue?
2. Difficulty remembering things or difficulty thinking clearly?
3. Increased back pain or aching joints?
4. Lack of interest in sex?
5. Increased urinary frequency?
6. Apathy or feeling that you just don't care?
7. Gain in weight, especially around your middle?
8. Increased irritability or uncontrolled anger?
9. Difficulty achieving and maintaining an erection?
10. Decreased enjoyment of life?
11. Increased anxiety or panic attacks?
12. Decreased muscle mass or strength?

Do you: (count 1 point for each "yes" answer)

1. Drink more than seven alcoholic beverages a week?
2. Have a history of significant testicular trauma or testicular cancer?

3. Take more than three pharmaceuticals regularly?

4. Have elevated cholesterol, triglycerides, or fasting blood sugar?

Scoring:

0–10 Congratulations, it looks like you aren't experiencing many symptoms; however, just because you are currently asymptomatic doesn't mean that your hormone levels are optimal. Maintaining healthy hormone function will be protective against metabolic syndrome, prostate cancer, and heart disease. Get your hormones tested now (see resource section) so you have a baseline established for the future. "You don't know where you are in your life, unless you know where you have been." —Dr. Meletis

11–20 It looks like you are beginning to have some problems and it's likely that you are suffering from sub-optimal testosterone. Being proactive and addressing this problem before it becomes debilitating is advised. You must get your hormones tested. If you determine it is your hormones, work with your doctor. If it is not your hormones, keep looking. Don't settle for mediocrity, you are too young to feel this old. Check out www.hischangeoflife.com for testing resources.

20–30 Your symptoms are indicative of significant hormone imbalance. Proper testing and treatment is recommended. You may not even remember what it's like to feel "normal" anymore!

30+ Wow, you could really use a boost! It looks like your hormones are pretty imbalanced, and are dramatically affecting your health and quality of life.

There have been several questionnaires developed to assess gonadal function, (gonads are reproductive organs, i.e., ovaries and testes). Certainly, none of them compare to measuring free testosterone levels through a trustworthy lab, but here is one example of a quick survey you can do to assess your risk of low testosterone. This questionnaire is really just to give you an idea of where you may stand; it's not designed to give you a diagnosis. Regardless of how you scored here, don't leave your health to chance or wait for your symptoms to get worse or new symptoms to appear. We know that your hormone levels are going to be falling automatically as you get older, but as you'll find out soon, there are many other factors that can exacerbate the situation. We recommend you get a comprehensive hormone panel that includes testosterone, DHEA, cortisol, estradiol, and progesterone levels. Men and women have the same hormones in their bodies; obviously, men should have higher levels of androgens and women higher levels of estrogen. There's a reason why men have a different ratio of hormones in their bodies, and if you are out of relative balance, it can wreak havoc on your body. Think of it this way: you are like a Corvette, and you require 92 octane fuel to keep your motor running at peak performance, but lately you have been trying to run on 87 octane gas. No wonder you are just plugging through life in the "slow lane" most of the time. Your engine won't run well enough to let you go full throttle. It's time to restore your performance to the best it can be.

NOTES

1. Mulligan T., Frick M.F., Zuraw Q.C., Stemhagen A., McWhirter C., "Prevalence of hypogonadism in males aged at least 45 years: the HIM study," *Int J Clin Pract.* (2006): Jul;60(7):762–9.

2. Hall, PhD, Susan A.; Andre B. Araujo, PhD; Gretchen R. Esche, MS; Rachel E. Williams, PhD; Richard V. Clark, MD, PhD; Thomas G. Travison, PhD; John B. McKinlay, PhD, "Treatment of symptomatic androgen deficiency results from the Boston Area Community Health Survey," *Arch Intern Med* (2008): 168(10):1070–1076.

3. Hall, S.A., G.R. Esche, A.B. Aroujo, T.G. Travison, R.V. Clark, R.E. Williams, J.B. McKinlay, "Correlates of low testosterone and symptomatic androgen deficiency in a population-based sample," *J Clin Encodrin Metab*, (2008) July 29.

4. Genesis 25: 1–6.

5. http://www.surgery.org/download/2007QFacts.pdf.

CHAPTER 3

The Role of Testosterone in the Male Body

Where exactly does testosterone come from and what does it do? What do you think of when you think of testosterone? Some people picture The Hulk with his muscles bulging out of his shirt and a temper that leads to destruction and decimation. Some of you may simply associate testosterone with sex drive, or maybe with puberty; you may think of it exclusively as the substance that helped you grow hair where there wasn't any and changed your voice so you didn't sound so much like your sister. We hope by now you have an idea that this hormone's affect on your body is much more complex and far-reaching than this, but let's start from the beginning. This chapter is kind of a "Get to Know Your Hormones: where do they come from and what do they do?" Some of this stuff can be a little tedious, but bear with us because it's important to understand the way things are designed to work so we can talk about some of the potential problems later.

Testosterone is a steroid hormone, which means that its chemical structure is similar to that of cholesterol. In fact, the body even uses cholesterol in the synthesis of testosterone. This will be an important fact to remember in a little while when we talk about cholesterol levels and cardiovascular health as it relates to hormone levels. If cholesterol levels are lowered too much, it may have an effect on total hormone levels since there is a deficit of starting material and this can dramatically affect your overall health. This is of particular danger with the use of cholesterol-lowering drugs that artificially bring total cholesterol levels down below even the bottom end of the reference range. Whenever we shift the balance of things within the body, there is always an indirect or unintended effect. Testosterone is also classified as an androgen, which is just a term to describe any substance, natural or synthetic, that influences the development of masculine secondary sex characteristics. Androgens are anabolic, which means that they promote protein production and the buildup of tissues (also called anabolism)

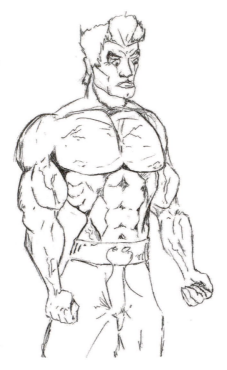

Figure 3.1 For many people the mention of
testosterone brings to mind the image of an
angry, muscle bound body builder.

instead of protein and tissue breakdown, which is called catabolism. This is why
they have been used historically in athletes who are trying to bulk up. So you may
hear testosterone referred to as a steroid, an androgen, or an anabolic hormone.
These words are describing three different characteristics about the hormone.

Small amounts of testosterone are produced in the adrenal cortex in both
men and women. The thecal cells of the ovaries and the placenta also produce
testosterone in women, but the majority of all testosterone is produced in the testes
of men. In fact, men typically produce about 12 to 20 times more testosterone
than women. A recent study that used mass spectrometry and gas chromatography
to measure testosterone production levels in men and women found that men
produce between 1.5 and 5.9 mg of testosterone per day, while women produce
only 0.3 to 0.5 mg/day.[1] More specifically, it is the interstitial or Leydig cells
in the testes that produce testosterone. The Leydig cells constitute almost 20
percent of the mass of the adult testes, though they are almost nonexistent during
childhood and they decrease in number significantly with aging. The hormone is
secreted into the blood where it acts locally on the Sertoli cells, another type of
cell present in the testes whose purpose is to govern the development of the sperm
cells. Sertoli cells are sometimes called "nurse cells" because they are responsible
for providing the developing spermatozoa with the proper nutrients that they
will need to develop into the fully "matured" sperm that are ready for their long

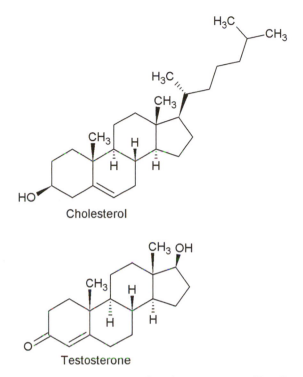

Cholesterol

Testosterone

Figure 3.2 You can see that the testosterone, like all steroid hormones, get its ring structure from cholesterol.

"quest for the holy ovum (egg)." While some testosterone is acting locally to help with this process, the majority of it leaves the testes and travels to tissues around the body. Most of it is bound to a transport protein called sex hormone binding globulin (SHBG). Before we get to where all of that testosterone is going, let's start from the very beginning. We want to explain a little about how the Leydig cells know to produce testosterone in the first place.

Our bodies use both electricity and chemicals to communicate between different cells, organs, and systems. One of the links between the nervous

You may think of the hypothalamus as the CEO of the company who reads over the reports from the investors, assesses the sales forecasts, and advises the management team on what steps need to be taken. The pituitary plays the role of the management team that takes direction from the CEO and delegates the work to the employees. The management team, like the pituitary, uses various communications to advise different employees to make whatever product they are assigned to produce, just as the pituitary tells the Sertoli cells to produce sperm and the Leydig cells to produce testosterone and the thyroid to produce thyroid hormone and the adrenal gland to produce cortisol, etc.

system (which transmits electrical impulses) and the endocrine system (which secretes chemical messengers that travel through the circulatory system) is the hypothalamus. Located just below the thalamus in your brain (and aptly named for that fact), the hypothalamus is the region of your brain that controls many metabolic processes. Think of it like the thermostat for your body, but in addition to controlling your temperature (which it does), it also controls your thirst, hunger, sexual appetite, hormone levels, and more. This is primarily done through the stimulus of the pituitary gland, which is often referred to as the master gland. The pituitary gland protrudes off of the bottom of the hypothalamus. The hypothalamus and the pituitary gland work so closely together that they are often referred to as the hypothalamic-pituitary (H-P) axis and described as a single system. They can be compared to the CEO (Chief Executive Officer) and COO (Chief Operations Officer) of a large corporation, which is not too farfetched since your body is comprised of 75 trillion cells (employees).

This system controls many different functions in the body, hence the nickname "master gland." However, for simplification purposes, we will focus on just the functions relating to the eventual production of testosterone and other sex hormones and forget about the many other purposes of the pituitary for now. The H-P system works like this: the hypothalamic neurons release a secretion called gonadotropin releasing hormone (GnRH) which travels down a vein to reach the anterior pituitary. Some of the cells in the anterior pituitary are stimulated by the GnRH to release luteinizing hormone (LH) and follicle stimulating hormone (FSH) into the blood stream. The LH and the FSH travel through the blood to the testes where the LH stimulates testosterone production in the Leydig cells, and the FSH stimulates spermatogenesis (sperm production) in the Sertoli cells. The whole process is governed by a negative feedback loop,

The SHBG protein binds to estrogen as well as testosterone, but has a greater affinity for testosterone. When either hormone is bound to SHBG, it becomes unavailable to target tissues. The protein-hormone complex cannot bind to receptors and therefore isn't biologically active.

Let's see if this helps: A basketball team has how many players on the court at a time? Five, right? And in a good man-on-man defense, those players aren't very "available" to score. It isn't until they break away (are not bound to) their defensive player that they are effective. Imagine if there wasn't a five-player limit on offense. If you could add a sixth man to the court, there wouldn't be a defensive player available to guard him, leaving him open. This is why it's important to test free testosterone levels and not just total levels. You could have adequate total testosterone levels, yet if all of that testosterone is bound to SHBG, it's not available to "score." Of course, hormones aren't exactly like basketball, there's no equivalent to a zone defense in this example, but I think you get the picture!

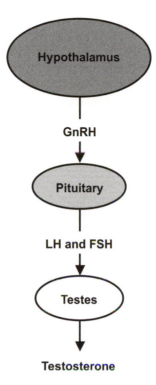

Figure 3.3 The Chain of Command.

which means that when there is enough testosterone in the bloodstream, it has a (down-regulating) effect on its own production. This is a necessary mechanism; otherwise, the testosterone production would be like an out-of-control locomotive: there would be no stopping it until it crashed. The hypothalamus senses the testosterone levels and reduces its output of GnRH, which reduces the release of LH, which, in turn, reduces the production of testosterone and so on and so forth. Whew! Are you still with us?

The hypothalamus' sensitivity to testosterone changes. For example, before the onset of puberty, it is very sensitive to low levels of the hormone, so there is very little GnRH released. During puberty, the sensitivity of the hypothalamus is dulled, resulting in an increase in GnRH and subsequently boosted testosterone levels. There is some evidence to support the theory that this change in sensitivity of the hypothalamus may be triggered by leptin (a small peptide hormone that controls appetite and satiety) and is prompted by a specific body size, rather than age. Now, we may be boring you with the names of all of these hormones, but this feedback loop and the changing sensitivity of the hypothalamus to circulating hormone levels are important to understand, as it will play a big part in later chapters when we discuss aging and changing hormone levels. It may also be noted that this GnRH–LH/FSH system works similarly in women by stimulating the ovaries to produce estrogen, which in turn influences the hypothalamus through a negative feedback loop.

Once the testosterone has been produced, it travels in the bloodstream mostly bound to the SHBG that is produced in the liver. There is an additional amount of the hormone bound to serum albumin (another protein) and a very tiny amount traveling in the blood that is not bound to a carrier protein. It is this "free" or unbound portion of the hormone that is able to interact with the receptors in the tissues and is referred to as biologically active testosterone or free testosterone. The SHBG is a way of regulating the hormone levels. When SHBG levels are high, it binds to more of the testosterone and leaves less of it to be effective in target tissues. Other hormones also bind to SHBG; as is indicated by its name, it carries the sex hormones estrogen and progesterone as well. As men age, not only do they produce less testosterone, but they produce more SHBG, so an even smaller percentage of their testosterone is able to affect tissues. When hormone levels are monitored in the blood, they often test for total testosterone (which would include the free as well as SHBG-bound testosterone) and test the SHBG levels. The free testosterone levels can then be calculated from this information. Other testing methods include salivary testing which only detects free hormone levels, as the carrier proteins are too large to pass into the saliva from the blood. There will be many more details on hormone testing. We'll get to it soon enough, but let's finish the story of testosterone first.

> Puberty is the sickest joke God plays on us. So you're just noticing members of the opposite sex: "Girls, girls, ooh." Naturally you want to look your best, and God says, "No! You will look the worst you've ever looked in your life!"—Eddie Izzard (comedian)

Though puberty is when we think of sex hormones making their debut, there are several times when sex hormone levels change to affect our development. Testosterone is what causes a developing baby to form a penis and scrotum instead of a clitoris and a vagina.

The male fetus begins secreting testosterone around the seventh week and, interestingly enough, if the testes are removed from an unborn animal at this stage, the animal will develop female sex organs even though it has male DNA. Similarly, if testosterone is supplied to a developing human female baby during this time, it will form male sexual organs. You may have thought it was just your Y chromosome that made you a man, but, as, it turns out, it starts with your testosterone! Testosterone is also what is responsible for the descent of the testicles into the scrotum during the final trimester of gestation. Testosterone levels are higher in the male fetus and continue to be higher than in females for approximately ten weeks after birth. It is speculated that this may have something to do with development of the male brain. And, of course, there's puberty. Who could forget that time when hormone levels surge and our bodies changed from those of children into adults? Let's face it, before puberty there isn't much of a difference between the bodies of little girls and little boys with the exception of genitalia. During this time of puberty, our bodies develop what we call secondary sex characteristics. In males, this is mostly due to, you guessed it, testosterone. First, we start noticing hair growth in the pubic area, upward to the umbilicus, on the face, and on the chest or back. Eventually, testosterone will decrease the growth of hair on the top of the head, while continuing to encourage it elsewhere. Testosterone causes enlargement of the penis, scrotum, and testes as well as elongation of the vocal cords, causing the voice to deepen. Testosterone also contributes to an increased testicular tone as well as increased production of sperm and increased fertility. Along with these more desired manly traits, the body odor changes, skin becomes thicker, and the increased secretion of sebum by the sebaceous glands causes acne, one of the hallmarks of puberty that many of us remember with abhorrence.

We mentioned before that androgens are anabolic, which means that they encourage proliferation of tissue, and testosterone is responsible for the increase in muscle mass that occurs during puberty that ultimately results in men having an average of 50 percent more muscle mass than women.[2] The anabolic effect takes place on bone as well, and the increase in circulating testosterone causes a deposition of calcium salts and thickening of bones, resulting in a greatly decreased incidence of osteoporosis among men compared to women. The testosterone surge also has an effect on the shape of bones, specifically causing the pelvis to narrow and lengthen into a funnel-like shape instead of the broad ovoid shape of a female pelvis. Are you still there? Had enough of this walk down memory lane? We know what you are thinking, "Sure testosterone helped shape me into the man I am, but what has it done for me lately?"

Just as it was responsible for initialing increasing muscle mass and strengthening bone during formative growth periods, testosterone is also in charge of maintaining muscle mass and bone strength throughout adulthood. Men with decreased testosterone levels have a greater incidence of osteoporosis and are at a much greater risk of fracture. Testosterone levels

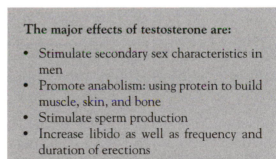

The major effects of testosterone are:

- Stimulate secondary sex characteristics in men
- Promote anabolism: using protein to build muscle, skin, and bone
- Stimulate sperm production
- Increase libido as well as frequency and duration of erections
- Reduce cardiovascular disease
- Increase energy and vigor
- Stimulate metabolism

affect cardiovascular health, not just by creating stronger heart muscle tissue, but also by altering cholesterol and triglyceride levels and controlling blood pressure. Testosterone replacement therapy in men **who are deficient** has been shown to raise red blood cell count, lower LDL cholesterol, decrease central fat, and increase muscle mass. Recent studies have also shown that testosterone acts as a calcium channel blocker, can be used to treat angina, and that men with coronary artery disease have lower testosterone levels than men without coronary artery disease.[3] It has recently been discovered that androgens increase neuron regeneration in rats with brain damage.[4] Studies have shown that testosterone may have a protective effect against Alzheimer's disease, and may even be beneficial in treatment for the condition.[5] It is often through studying the effects of testosterone on the disease processes of men with lower-than-normal testosterone levels that we can gain a greater understanding of the extensive role hormones play in regulating our body's systems.

The presence of testosterone in the testicles is important to the Sertoli cells, which nurture the sperm cells through development, but remember that the primary stimulation of sperm production comes from the pituitary in the form of FSH. This hormone prompts the Sertoli cells to produce sperm much like the LH prompts the production of testosterone. Testosterone plays a more important role in libido as well as the frequency and duration of erections, system is the which, as you can imagine, can affect fertility. Low libido is the symptom that most often prompts physicians to test for testosterone in both men and women. It seems that decreased libido as well as impaired ability to obtain an erection is occurring with much greater frequency. Remember when Bob Dole made erectile dysfunction (ED) a household phrase? Do you think that men have suddenly developed a Viagra® deficiency? It's possible that we have suffered from the same symptoms of sexual dysfunction for years and the only difference is that it's become more socially acceptable to discuss in both private and public forums. Another possibility is that our chronic stress levels, chronic diseases, and environmental influences, coupled with a lack of attention to hormone health, have led us into a sexual slump. The truth is probably a combination of these two factors. The little blue pill and the drugs similar to it only address part of the problem: the erection. Many men find that not only do they have trouble getting and maintaining an erection, but that they just aren't "in the mood" as often. As you can imagine, this change in interest can cause a lot of problems and confusion in an otherwise healthy marriage. And healthy testosterone levels in women are also involved in sexual appetite, so the problem can be related to hormones on both sides. As we know, it takes two to tango, or not to as the case may be. Remember, guys, there is a BIG difference (no pun intended) between getting by and really feeling alive. Don't just settle for punching in and out each day. It is time to THRIVE, not just survive.

Let us explain a little about what happens biologically behind the scenes during sexual stimulation for men. The autonomic nervous system is the part of our nervous system that is responsible for the things we don't think about. Think of it as controlling functions that occur automatically (breathing), as opposed to those we have to think about (moving your hand). There are two main divisions of the autonomic nervous system: the parasympathetic system is the "rest and digest" system that plays a role when you are relaxing, and the sympathetic system is the "fight-or-flight" system that kicks into gear when you need a quick response. The parasympathetic nervous system is dominant during times when your body is calm and focusing its resources on systems such as reproduction, digestion, urination, and defecation and is responsible for erections. The sympathetic system is dominant when you are stressed. It shunts your blood away from your digestive center and into your large muscles to provide energy and oxygen for moving quickly, and causes your heart to beat faster and your bronchial passages to dilate to provide more oxygen to the tissues. The sympathetic system should be used in short spurts for emergent situations. Again, it is the parasympathetic system that is responsible for erections, which explains why it is difficult to achieve and maintain an erection when you are nervous or anxious.

Anxiety tells the body that there is a danger and triggers the sympathetic nervous system, which takes over and shunts blood where it is most needed. And in terms of systems required for immediate survival, the penis is pretty low on the totem pole. During an erection, the parasympathetic nervous system causes the release of nitric oxide into the corpus cavernosum

> Don West, pharmacist at Lloyd Center Compounding pharmacy in Portland, OR, told us that he has seen an increase in hormone prescriptions for men over the last several years, and gives credit to the ED drugs such as Viagra® for opening up the dialog and making it more acceptable for men to discuss and seek treatment for their problems.

of the penis. The corpus cavernosum are the sponge-like erectile tissues along the shaft of the penis that fill with blood during an erection. The nitric oxide is produced by enzymes called nitric oxide synthases, which are stimulated by testosterone.[6] The nitric oxide (NO) stimulates an enzyme called guanylate cyclase, which results in an increased level of cyclic guaniosine monophosphate (cGMP). The cGMP causes vasodilation in the intimal cushions of the penis, which causes blood to pool in the corpus cavernosa, resulting in an erection. At the end of an erection, another enzyme called cGMP-specific phosphodiesterase type 5 (PDE5) is responsible for the degradation of the cGMP in the corpus cavernosum which allows the blood vessels to constrict and the blood to exit the penis. Sympathetic stimulation also causes constriction of these blood vessels, preventing them from filling with blood. This process is important to understand because it is how ED drugs like Viagra® work. Viagra® (sildenafil) has a molecular structure that is similar to cGMP, and it binds to and blocks the action of the PDE5, causing the cGMP to be active longer than it would be otherwise. Testosterone levels have been shown to increase production of nitric oxide in animal studies.[7] Nitric oxide then stimulates the production of cGMP causing the same vasodiltation and erection. Just in case your eyes are crossed from all of that technical talk, basically what we're saying is that testosterone stimulates the production of nitric oxide which causes the blood vessels in your penis to relax and fill with blood, causing an erection. Your penis holds 8 to 10 times more blood when it is erect compared to when it's flaccid. Essentially, erectile dysfunction pharmaceuticals work by keeping the nitric oxide around longer so the blood stays pooled longer. Healthy testosterone levels increase the release of nitric oxide naturally, and you don't have to plan ahead to make sure you are ready for the big occasion.

So, maybe you don't need the little pill after all; it is time to look at the BIG-GER picture. You may be thinking, what's the difference then if supplementing testosterone does the same thing as Viagra® by increasing the amount of cGMP? The difference is this: testosterone is a substance that is normally present in your body. Men with normal levels of testosterone shouldn't need a magic blue pill. The goal here is to achieve and maintain normal levels of testosterone (physiological levels), not increase levels beyond the normal healthy range. The normal blood level of Viagra® is, of course, none at all! So, if you are thinking about surrendering and getting a little pill as a helper, you may want to look at the real reason behind the problem. And don't just chalk it up to old age . . . get your hormone levels tested and address the underlying cause. Normalizing your testosterone levels should also prevent the lack of libido or sexual appetite that many men suffer from and that Viagra,® Cialis,® and Levitra® fail to address. And they can't solve the other symptoms of low testosterone—remember them?—fatigue, breast enlargement, decreased muscle mass, mood swings, depression. As I (C. Meletis) shared in my book, Better Sex Naturally,[8] your sex performance is a reflection of your overall health. It can serve as a barometer of health changes or as an indicator of stability.

Just as nitric oxide induces vasodilation in the penis during the production of an erection, it can also induce the same effect in all blood vessels, and, through this mechanism, testosterone plays an integral part of controlling blood pressure. Testosterone can induce nitric oxide in the endothelial cells (the cells that line the blood vessels) throughout the body. Of course, enabling erections is important, but controlling blood pressure by maintaining healthy testosterone levels could prevent heart disease, the number one cause of death in men and women. If you think of your heart and your blood vessels as a "container" that holds your blood, you can imagine that when your arteries and veins become rigid or constricted it decreases the size of that container. The volume of your blood should more or less stay the same. So you can imagine that if you decrease the size of the container (but not the volume of the contents) that the pressure would increase.

Increased blood pressure puts a lot of stress on the heart as well as the walls of the blood vessels and can lead to heart failure or aneurisms. Aneurisms occur when areas of the arteries are weak and rupture. Nitric oxide, and by proxy testosterone, plays in important role in allowing the blood vessels to dilate, which decreases the pressure, like increasing the size of a container while keeping the same volume of contents. Though many people may just be realizing that hormones play such a large role in the health of men, The Journal of Hypertension published an article describing the relationship between testosterone and blood pressure 20 years ago![9] They found an inverse relationship between blood pressure and testosterone levels, meaning that the men with high blood pressure had lower testosterone levels and vice versa. Well, it's never too late to start applying this information that has been "lying around" all this time.

Testosterone and other androgen hormones have receptors in the liver, and when they bind to those receptors, they induce the synthesis of triglyceride lipase, an enzyme that breaks down triglycerides to be absorbed and used by the body for energy. Translation: testosterone literally helps you break down fat. The liver will also decrease its production of SHBG, cortisol binding globulin (CBG), and thyroxin-binding globulin (TBG) in the presence of testosterone. These proteins are used to transport their respective hormones in the blood, and by decreasing the production of the transport proteins, there is an increase in the available forms of these hormones to the tissues. Therefore, the net effect is that testosterone actually increases the availability of more testosterone, cortisol, and thyroid hormone to tissues.

In the kidney, androgens such as testosterone stimulate the production of erythropoietin, which is a hormone that controls red blood cell production. Therefore, testosterone increases hematocrit (red blood cell count). In fact, this is one thing that should be monitored during testosterone supplementation, as you don't want your hematocrit to increase too much. Testosterone levels modulate the immune system by inhibiting T suppressor cell function which improves the immune system's ability to respond to an attack and also helps to mitigate auto-immune diseases by reducing the titers of antinuclear antibodies (these are your body's immune cells that have mistakenly attacked your own cells). This mechanism likely accounts for at least part of the reason why autoimmune diseases such as lupus and multiple sclerosis are so much more prevalent in women compared to men.[10]

Testosterone, testosterone, testosterone. So far, all we have talked about is testosterone. What about the other hormones? There are several other androgens worth mentioning: dihydrotestosterone (DHT), dehydroepiandrosterone (DHEA), androstenedione, and androstenediol. Many of these hormones exist as precursors or metabolites of testosterone and estrogen. In fact, it's hard to talk about any of these hormones without taking into account the effects of others because the body can change them from one thing into another. One of the major ways that testosterone influences the male body is actually through its conversion into estrogen! Before we get into that, let's go over these other androgens.

- **Dehyroepiandrosterone (DHEA)**—produced from cholesterol in the adrenal cortex, this hormone is both a primary precursor to all sex hormones and a stress hormone. DHEA has the ability to enhance immune resistance;[11] reduce risk of cancer,[12] coronary artery disease, and osteoporosis; improve blood sugar,[13] facilitate weight loss, and help control Alzheimers' disease. DHEA is often touted as a drug to help people age more gracefully.[14] It is currently available over the counter; however, because it is a precursor to other sex hormones, supplementation should be monitored as it could raise estrogen or testosterone to unhealthy levels.
- **Androstenedione**—an androgenic steroid that is produced by the testes, the adrenal cortex, and the ovaries. Androstenedione is produced from DHEA and is a parent structure to estrogen as well as testosterone. This substance has been banned by the International Olympic Committee and other sporting organizations for use as an athletic or bodybuilding supplement.

- **Androstenediol**—a direct metabolite of DHEA, has about 1/475th the androgenic power of testosterone. One form of androstenediol is an immune stimulant; it induces production of white blood cells and platelets.
- **Androsterone**—created in the liver during the breakdown of androgens, it has been used as a pheromone, but there is little data to support this. The chemical structure is similar to estrone, and it can be found in approximately equal amounts in the plasma and urine of men and women.
- **Dihydrotestosterone (DHT)**—produced in the adrenal cortex, the prostate, the testes, and the hair follicles, this hormone is another metabolite of testosterone, but is a more potent androgen than testosterone. An enzyme called 5-alpha reductase is responsible for the conversion of testosterone to DHT, and, once converted, it binds more strongly to androgen receptors than testosterone itself. DHT has been implicated as the primary contributing factor in male pattern baldness as well as benign prostatic hyperplasia (BPH) which is a process where the prostate becomes enlarged. Higher-than-average levels of the 5-alpha reductase have been found in the scalp, inducing elevated DHT levels, which induce the formation of fine, short, non-pigmented hairs. We don't think we need to draw the correlation between androgen levels and acne, as you probably learned this one firsthand during high school, but DHT is active in sebaceous glands producing sebum that can clog pores and cause acne. Unlike testosterone, DHT cannot be converted to estrogen, so its effects are exclusively through androgenic receptors. DHT also plays a role in the formation of many male sex characteristics both *in utero* and in puberty.

There are several ways that testosterone and other androgens have an effect on the body. The first is to bind to testosterone receptors in target tissues, as is mentioned above when we were talking about DHT. Because DHT has a stronger affinity for said receptors, it has several times the androgen affect that testosterone has. DHT is not converted to estrogen so it has no effect on estrogen receptors.

As you can see from the hormone pathways, testosterone (in addition to most of the other androgens) can easily be converted to estrogen and, through this mechanism, exerts many effects on the body. Some of these effects are necessary and include the closing of epiphyseal plates (areas of bone growth found in long bones in the body) to conclude growth. This is one of the reasons why women stop growing at an earlier age than men, because they have greater concentration of estrogen. The conversion of testosterone into estradiol is governed by an aromatase enzyme and occurs mainly in the liver, brain, and fat tissue. Therefore, increased fat can lead to increased estrogen levels. Remember that testosterone is responsible for the creation of muscle, and, therefore, as more of the testosterone is converted to estrogen that means there is less testosterone to stimulate muscle growth and more estrogen to promote fat storage. Increased fat tissue helps to convert more testosterone to estrogen and so on and so forth. It's a downward

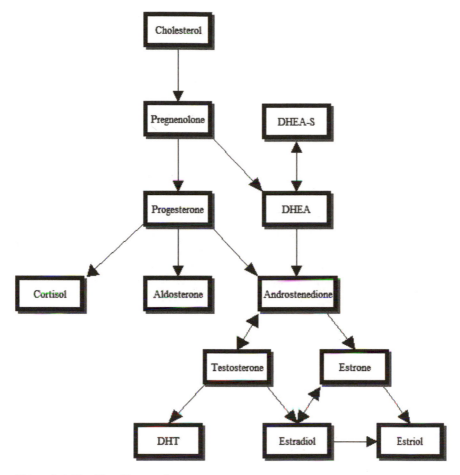

Figure 3.4 The Steroid cascade.

spiral in which many men find themselves stuck. Estrogen levels decline in women as they age, but increase in men due primarily to this cycle with aromatase. As estrogen levels rise, the estrogen stimulates more SHBG to be produced, but remember that the SHBG prefers testosterone, so it binds to what little testosterone is left, leaving an even smaller amount free to affect the tissues. In this way, the SHBG amplifies the effects of the estrogen by stealing even more of the testosterone from the picture.

By now you should be pretty familiar with testosterone and what it SHOULD be doing in your body. Of course, *should* is the optimal word here. As we've covered, the body's road to testosterone production is long and complicated, and the effects that the hormone has on the body are diverse and far-reaching. The real point is, there are MANY places that this ideal system can run into problems. There are many effects of imbalanced testosterone levels, and too much or too little of the hormone can create and contribute to considerable health problems, as you've already gotten a glimpse of. The next chapter will go over some of the most common and significant effects of imbalanced testosterone levels and chances are many of them will sound all too familiar. But never fear, shortly we will be telling you what you can do to take back your youth or keep this all from happening to you!

NOTES

1. *The Journal of Clinical Endocrinology & Metabolism*, 82:5, 1492–1496.

2. Vierhapper, H., P. Nowotny, and W. Waldhäusl, "Determination of testosterone production rates in men and women using stable isotope/dilution and mass spectrometry1, *Reproductive Endocrinology*.

3. English, K.M., O. Mandour, R.P. Steeds, M.J. Diver, T.H. Jones, K.S. Channer, "Men with coronary artery disease have lower levels of androgens than men with normal coronary angiograms," *Eur Heart J* (2000): 21:890–4.

4. Z.K., L. Shen, H. Ke, F. Li, L.M. Ni, Q. H. Li, "Effects of androgen on the expression of brain aromatase cytopigment and nerve growth factor in neonatal rats with hypoxic-ischemic brain damage," *Zhongguo Dang Dai Er Ke Za Zhi* (2008) Aug;10(4):441–6.

5. University of Southern California, "Testosterone therapy may prevent Alzheimer's disease," *Science Daily* (2006) Dec 20 pg ?

6. Traish, A, and N. Kim. "The physiological role of androgens in penile erection: regulation of corpus cavernosum structure and function," *J Sex Med* (2005) Nov;2(6): 759–70.

7. Du, J., and E.M. Hull, Department of Psychology, "Effects of testosterone on neuronal nitric oxide synthase and tyrosine hydroxylase," *Brain Res* (1999) Jul 31; 836(1–2): 90–8.

8. Meletis C., S.M. Fitzgerald, "*Better Sex Naturally*" Harper Collins, 1999.

9. Khaw K., and E. Barrett-Connor, "Blood pressure and endogenous testosterone in men: an inverse relationship," *Journ of Hyperten* (1988) 6:329–332.

10. Gamineri, A., R. Pasquali, J. Endocrinol, "Testosterone therapy in men: Clinical and pharmacological perspectives," *Invest* (2000) 23:196–214.

11. Straub, R. et al, "Serum DHEA and DHEA sulfate are negatively correlated with serum interleukin-6 (IL-6), and DHEA inhibits IL-6 secretion from mononuclear cells in man in vitro," *J Clin Endocrino. Metab* (1998) 83:2012–17. Daynes, R.K. and B. Araneo, "Natural regulators of T-cell lymphokine production in vivo," *J Immunother* (1992) 12: 174–79.

12. Rudman, D., et al, "Plasma dehydroepiandrosterone sulfate in nursing home men," *J Ann Geriatr Soc* (1990) 38:421–27.

13. Bates, G., et al, "DEA attenuates study induced declines in insulin sensitivity in postmenopausal women," *Ann NY Acad Sci* (1995) 774:291–3.

14. Zenk, J., *Living Longer in the Boomer Age*, (New York: Advanced Research Press, 1998).

CHAPTER 4

Health Risks of Low or High Testosterone

You should be starting to get the picture about the roles that testosterone plays in the body as well as its complex interaction with other hormones. We hope you also understand that it's important for us to monitor our hormone levels because there are so many things that can affect them. We have touched upon some of the effects of low testosterone when we were exploring all of its purposes in the body because so many of the studies have been modeled that way. We often discover the role that testosterone plays due to its tested deficiency and then its effects on a given condition when administered. Next, we are going to further explore some of the health risks of having low testosterone levels, and then what happens if the levels are too high. If we could pick one word of all the thousands in this book to stress most it would be **balance**. The whole point here is the importance of **balancing** hormone levels. Just as there are many effects and risks of low testosterone levels, there are similar dangers with levels that are too high and we are not advocating for levels higher than would be found in your body under optimal conditions, as hormone levels that are too high (as well as too low) can lead to many health complications.

So what kind of problems do we expect to see in men with measured low hormone levels? Well, now that you have a better understanding of all of the roles that testosterone plays in the body, you can easily imagine that the effects of its absence are far-reaching and varied. Andropause isn't an official medical diagnosis, but falls into the broader category of hypogonadism that is caused simply from aging. Hypogonadism is defined as an underperformance of the gonads, or in the case of men, the testes. As we've learned, the two main products of the testes are sperm and testosterone. Hypogonadism can cause low sperm count and infertility, but for the sake of this book we are more interested in the underproduction of testosterone. Hypogonadism can be caused by several different factors. It can be congenital, meaning you were born with the issue and for various reasons there are never enough sex hormones produced. It can be surgical as in the case of castration, which is an uncommon practice in modern society, but has a long history in many cultures for social, religious, and political reasons. And, of course, hypogonadism can be caused by disease processes, infection, injury, lifestyle, and age. It is the latter causes of this condition that we are most concerned with, as these are factors that we can control. However, for the purposes of understanding the effects of low testosterone, it doesn't matter what the cause is.

Some of the many consequences a lack of testosterone can produce are already well understood by the general public, especially if we look to our treatment of livestock and other animals whose endocrine system isn't all that different from our own. For example, I (S. Wood) was visiting a friend who lives in a rural area of central Louisiana. They have several young donkeys and has recently been having trouble with the male donkeys trying to mate with the females. The most common and effective way to curb this behavior, as well as ensure that they won't find themselves with several new donklets (actually called colts or foals just like horses), is to castrate or remove the testicles of the male donkeys. Of course this removes their ability to create sperm and thus to procreate, but it will also eventually remove their desire to do so. My weekend in Louisiana just happened to coincide with the visit from the vet, and I couldn't help but think of andropause as I witnessed this common farm procedure. Many animals are rendered sterile by similar means, and often for reasons that extend beyond the prevention of offspring. Castration is used to moderate aggression in many animals from hogs to bulls to pit bulls. It has even been used to control the behavior of criminals. In the 1930s and 1940s, many sex offenders were surgically castrated to prevent them from repeat offenses. A study in Germany in 1963 found that the recidivism rate (rate of repeated offense) of castrated sex offenders was 2.3 percent compared to 80 percent in the control group over a twenty-year period.[1] As the Louisiana vet explained to me, after several weeks those donkeys would lose interest and stop chasing the females around the pasture. Alright, enough about castration, we've probably got most of you cringing, so relax and let go of your beloved family jewels. We simply want make the point that we have known for decades the many effects of removing testosterone from the picture completely.

A healthy man can produce about 5 to 6 mg of testosterone daily, and the total blood level should be between 270 and 1,070 ng/dl (that's nanograms per deciliter, a unit of measurement that is used by the lab). As we will discuss in great detail later in this book, blood isn't always the best way to measure testosterone levels. Looking at free testosterone levels or those not bound to carrier proteins in the blood is a more accurate measurement of what is actually available to the tissues. It is possible for a man to have testosterone levels that are well within the desired range, yet still be experiencing symptoms of testosterone deficiency, if those hormones are all bound to the carrier protein SHBG and not available for the tissues to use. Decreased levels of testosterone are known to cause symptoms such as erectile dysfunction, decrease in muscle mass, fatigue, and difficulty concentrating.

A study that appeared in the *Archives of General Psychiatry* in March of 2008[2] showed that men with low **free** testosterone levels were 271 percent more likely to show signs of depression than men with normal testosterone levels. That's almost three times as likely! The study looked at almost 4,000 men from Australia who were screened for depression and compared the levels of free testosterone in their blood. Testosterone may increase the ability of the body to use serotonin and norepinephrine in the brain. The exact mechanism through which this is done is not yet understood—this may explain why depression is more prevalent among women during the first six decades of life—but the difference in occurrence becomes negligible later in life. The symptoms of depression are very similar to those of testosterone deficiency, so many men are diagnosed with depression and treated with anti-depressants when they complain to their doctors of fatigue, apathy, depression, irritability, and low libido. In most cases, testosterone levels are never even checked because the clinical effects of low testosterone are not well understood or commonly treated by most physicians.

The one symptom that does prompt many physicians to test for testosterone levels is low libido or lack of sex drive. In fact, this is the number one complaint that results in lab tests for testosterone levels in both men and women. Testosterone receptor sites are found throughout the body, including in the brain, blood vessels, and muscles. These tissues are "turned on" when testosterone binds to the receptors. Sexual arousal begins in the brain where testosterone ignites the neurons that signal for sexual stimulation and continues in other tissues. Without adequate levels of testosterone, the male's sex life is significantly affected both emotionally as well as physically. Studies have found that men with low testosterone not only suffer from a decreased libido, but impotence as well.[3] There was a time when erectile dysfunction (ED) wasn't discussed on prime-time TV commercials and simply remained something that neither men nor their wives talked about. This is still a sensitive topic for most men, despite its role in mainstream media and pop culture. If there is one good thing to come from pharmaceutical companies advertising their products to the general public on TV, it may be that it has opened up the dialog about sexual dysfunction in many households. It's a lot easier to talk about your personal difficulties when you know that more than 25 million men worldwide have taken Viagra.® It's getting easier to discuss, but just as the commercials often depict, most men go through a period where they think that what they are going through is unique to them, or at least believe that it doesn't happen to other men their age. Of course, men (and, by proxy, the women who love them) have been suffering from symptoms of erectile dysfunction since long before its two letter acronym was common terminology. Testosterone plays a significant role in libido as well as the achievement and maintenance of an erection. Animal studies have shown that exposure to testosterone increases the synthesis of nitric oxide in the vascular nerve endings of the corpora cavernosa in the penis.[4]

Though many men have a difficult time talking about their problems in this area of their lives to begin with, ultimately they are more likely to seek help for sexual dysfunction than they would be for many other parameters of their health. Let's face it, most men will suffer through the flu, deal with chronic back pain, and even ignore blood in their stool, but a change in their bedroom performance will lead them to look for some kind of treatment. Even when libido is decreased and they aren't in the mood as often, sex is usually important enough to most guys to motivate them to look into the problem. In fact, many men may talk to their doctors about problems of impotence initially and discover that, in fact, they are suffering from a number of ailments including those associated with metabolic syndrome and increased risk for heart disease.[5] The conditions of low testosterone levels, erectile dysfunction, and metabolic syndrome can be thought of as a trio of conditions that go hand in hand . . . in hand.[6]

Although there are many symptoms of androgen deficiency, metabolic syndrome may be the **single greatest health risk associated with low testosterone** levels because the presence of these risk factors significantly increases the likelihood of heart attack, stroke, and death. In fact, one journal recently called metabolic syndrome "the most important public health threat of the 21st Century." (Traish AM, 2008)

Low androgen levels don't just cause problems in the bedroom; decreased testosterone levels have been found in as many as 64 percent of men with diabetes.[7] In fact, low testosterone levels are so commonly found with symptoms of metabolic syndrome that they have been talked about as a specific entity: Hypoandrogen-metabolic syndrome (HAM)[8] and lab values indicating low testosterone levels can serve as an early warning of coming metabolic syndrome.[9] Metabolic syndrome is sometimes referred to as Syndrome X and is a name for a group of conditions that often occur together that increase your risk of heart disease, diabetes, and stroke. The conditions included in metabolic syndrome are high blood pressure, increased fat around the abdomen (or "apple shape",) abnormal cholesterol levels, increased triglyceride levels, and elevated insulin levels or insulin resistance, which is a pre-diabetic condition. Diabetes is truly an epidemic in this country and around the world. The National Institute of Diabetes and Digestive and Kidney Diseases estimates that over 23 million people ages 20 and older have diabetes. That's 7.8 percent of the population. It gets worse, as almost 26 percent of Americans over 20 had an impaired glucose tolerance test, a test that indicates a pre-diabetic state. If you look at people over the age of 60, that number jumps to 35.4 percent.[10] That's over one-third of people over the age of 60 that have a pre-diabetic condition!

Metabolic syndrome includes:
• Blood sugar dysregulation
• Elevated triglycerides
• Elevated LDL cholesterol
• Decreased HDL cholesterol
• Increased visceral fat
• Increased waist circumference
• High blood pressure

Studies show that restoring healthy physiological levels of testosterone can improve metabolic syndrome by reducing plasma cholesterol, increasing plasma high-density lipoprotein (HDL cholesterol, often referred to as "good cholesterol"), and decreasing waist circumference.[11] Normalizing testosterone levels can also decrease visceral fat (fat that is located inside the abdominal cavity around your organs).[12] The visceral fat cells respond to insulin differently than the "average" fat cells you find in the rest of the body. The receptors in these fat cells are much more likely to be insulin-resistant. This is a very powerful relationship; you can literally use testosterone to treat metabolic syndrome, as it will lower fasting glucose, fasting insulin levels, and glycosylated hemoglobin (HbA1c).[13] Of course, combining any therapy with exercise and proper diet is necessary, but testosterone deficiency is a known cause of metabolic syndrome.

Fat cells contain the enzyme aromatase that can convert testosterone into estrogen. Now, as we've said before, it is normal for men to have some estrogen in their bodies, but at higher levels, the estrogen causes a lot of problems including an increased risk of heart attack or stroke and increased risk of prostate cancer. Furthermore, the high estrogen levels can trick the brain into thinking that enough testosterone is being produced by saturating the receptors in the hypothalamus and activating the feedback mechanism to stop production. Estrogen also stimulates the production of SHBG, which binds to testosterone and lowers the available free testosterone levels. For this reason, we sometimes refer to SHBG as an estrogen amplifier because it downplays the effects of testosterone and increases the effects of estrogen. So, we have created a cycle that becomes hard to break: low testosterone = increased fat = more estrogen = lower testosterone.

"John" is a local professional who was trying to launch a new company, but was having a hard time making things happen because he was so fatigued. He couldn't focus or think clearly. He felt he was lucky that he had been at his current job for a couple of decades and could operate on autopilot, but problems arose when he tried to branch out with the new business. He confessed that he felt "like the walking dead." He was just going through the motions of living, literally punching in and out of his daily life like a factory worker punching in and out on a time clock. I diagnosed him with severe sleep apnea, and upon treatment he literally sprung back to life. His new company is moving forward and he thanks me each time we meet for giving his life back. The bottom line is he took his life back, he took my guidance, and basically told himself with the last bit of energy he had, "Heck no, I won't go without a fight." There is no question that we saved his life. We Eventually fine-tuned his treatment plan with some bio-identical testosterone as well, but treating the primary cause of his imbalance was critical to his success.

Increased fat and decreased muscle tone together don't just make you look worse; they can also contribute to significant fatigue. One of the ways they do this is by causing obstructive sleep apnea (OSA). Sleep apnea is a condition where there are significant pauses in breathing during sleep. This is most often caused by an obstruction in the airway. OSA typically goes hand in hand with snoring, and if you've ever slept in the room with someone who was a snorer, you may know that you can often hear their breathing stop for brief periods of time. There are many causes for apnea including recent orthodontic work, narrow jaw, big tongue, or thick neck. Many people have an increased incidence of OSA when they have been drinking, or have taken a sedative or sleep aid because the alcohol or medication causes the muscles in the airway to relax. We know that testosterone increases muscle tone, and in its absence the tissues in the back of the throat become flabby and untoned; they can sag and block the airway during sleep. You may see this cause an increase in snoring, but many of the effects are far more subtle. If this is happening to you, you may not realize that your body is waking hundreds of times a night gasping for air. You may not wake to the point of consciousness, but you are likely prevented from getting adequate restorative sleep.

How does a little snoring affect your testosterone levels? Sleep apnea affects how much oxygen your entire body is receiving, including the testicles. Lack of oxygen prevents the testicles from receiving the nourishment they need in order to produce adequate testosterone. The hypothalamus and pituitary are starved of oxygen as well, affecting their ability to effectively pass down "orders" for hormone production. In addition, the stress response caused by a lack of oxygen will further shut down blood supply to the testicles and other tissues that the body deems not critical during an acute stressful situation. Sleep apnea can cause hypogonadism and fatigue as well as hypertension, stroke, cardiac arrhythmia, diabetes, and more This is literally a catch-22; if you have low testosterone, you are more likely to have sleep apnea, but sleep apnea also causes low testosterone. In our clinical practices, we routinely see men with low testosterone levels that also have obstructive sleep apnea? The question must be asked, which came first, the low testosterone or sleep apnea. As with many of the biologic processes described in this book, the answer is not clear. What is clear is that this spiral, where low testosterone causes apnea which causes lowered testosterone, makes it even more important to address these issues before they continue to decline.

Remember the *Seinfeld* episode that talked about "The Manssiere" or "The Bro"? These were proposed names for a bra for men, or maybe you've joked with friends about moobs, short for man boobs. Many men find themselves with enough extra fat on their chest that it literally looks like they need a bra. Sometimes this is simply an effect of increased body fat all over the body. Yet, many times a hormone profile that is high in estrogen and low in testosterone will literally cause fat to be preferentially distributed to the breast area and cause an increase in the size of the mammary glands. In some cases, there can even be milk secretion. No, the clinical name for this condition isn't "mooby," it's actually called gynecomastia. In the case where there is just an excess of body fat, then the condition can be called pseudogynecomastia since the symptoms mimic increased mammary glands. Remember, increased body fat means that all of those fat cells are working to convert the testosterone that is present into estrogen, thereby exacerbating the problem. Don't worry, we're going to talk about how to mitigate this when we get to the treatment sections in later chapters. In fact, normalizing testosterone levels doesn't just decrease breast tissue. A study treated 60 healthy men with measured low testosterone levels by giving them transdermal testosterone. They found a significant increase in total body lean mass as well as skeletal muscle and a decrease in abdominal organ fat, which, as we know, translates into protection from metabolic syndrome and diabetes.[14]

As we said way back when we were first introducing you to testosterone, it is a steroid hormone like the other sex hormones, and these hormones are all produced from cholesterol. Cholesterol gets a pretty bad reputation in the modern era, but in fact it has many imperative roles in the body including maintaining proper cell membrane fluidity, the metabolism of fat soluble vitamins, involvement in cell signaling processes, and antioxidant properties. Perhaps most important for our purposes is cholesterol's role as a precursor to vitamin D and all steroid hormones including the sex hormones, cortisol, and aldosterone. Of course, just as we have advocated for the **balance** of testosterone and other hormones, it is important to keep cholesterol levels balanced as well.

The human body has some amazing ways to correct imbalances. One of the ways that our bodies will attempt to compensate for deficiencies is to increase quantities of a starting material needed to create whatever we are deficient in. In this situation, our bodies will increase production of cholesterol in response to low hormone levels. This is just one of the mechanisms where hypogonadism or andropause contributes to heart disease and metabolic syndrome. Testosterone stimulates the heart muscle to be lean and powerful and function optimally, just as it promotes lean muscle mass in the rest of the body. Studies have also shown an association between low testosterone levels and a higher occurrence of coronary artery disease and atherosclerosis.[15] Testosterone is cardioprotective and will protect the heart from damage due to loss of oxygen.[16] In fact, Michael Klentze, MD, PhD, of the Klentze Institute of Health Aging in Munich, Germany, reports that there are more testosterone receptors in the heart than in any other tissue in the body![17] In 2002, the *American Journal of Hypertension* published a correlation between low testosterone levels and high blood pressure. We learned during chapter 3 that testosterone increases the nitric oxide level in the penis and also in the blood vessels affecting blood pressure. We have seen some studies that suggest low testosterone levels are consistent with high LDL cholesterol (bad cholesterol). This may also lead to hardening of the blood vessels and rising blood pressure.

We mentioned previously that male sex hormones are anabolic. You may be familiar with this terminology as we've all heard about the performance-enhancing substances that many of our most revered athletic stars may (or may not) have used. From the Olympics and the Tour de France scandals to *The Mitchell Report*, these stories seem to be ubiquitous on ESPN, as well as network news. Remember, anabolic simply means that these hormones promote protein and muscle-building as opposed to breakdown. It is the lack of this anabolic effect that causes a decrease in muscle mass, thinning of skin, and osteoporosis in hypogonadal men. After the age of 60, the rate of hip fractures doubles every decade in men, and men with low testosterone levels are six times more likely to break a hip during a fall than men with normal levels.[18] Most studies where

Symptoms of decreased testosterone levels include:

- Erectile dysfunction
- Infertility
- Decrease in body hair
- Increase in body fat
- Decrease in muscle mass
- Development of breast tissue (gynecomastia)
- Loss of bone mass
- Fatigue
- Decreased sex drive
- Decreased mental acuity
- Hot flashes
- Irritability
- Depression
- Decreased flexibility
- Insulin resistance
- Increased risk of heart disease
- Premature death

testosterone is given to hypogonadal men have shown a significant increase in bone mineral density.[19] In other words, testosterone is responsible for building tissues: **muscles, skin, and bone**. When the levels are low, then we find that muscle mass decreases resulting in loss of strength, weakened bone density (which increases possibility of fracture), and thinner skin which causes more wrinkles and increased incidence of surface cuts or tears.

It goes without saying that the net effect of all of these conditions that low testosterone leads to or enables is an increased risk of death, and one study found just that. Doctors in Germany that followed 2,000 subjects found that men with low testosterone levels had more than 2.5 times the risk of dying during the next 10 years compared to men with higher, normal testosterone levels. They eliminated age, smoking history, alcohol habits, level of exercise, and waist measurement as factors and the risk was still 2.5 times greater! This study also found that those study subjects with low testosterone were more likely to have died from cancer or cardiovascular disease than the control group. This study essentially sums it all up and makes a sensational headline: "**Low testosterone = earlier death.**"[20] The body is complex, and the endocrine system is a perfect example. The higher mortality rate is probably a result of the increased incidence of heart disease and diabetes that we have mentioned earlier. The point here is that a hormone imbalance caused by environmental factors and age may be at the root of **many different symptoms**.

There is a time and place for a patch job. Even when you get a flat tire, you need a **temporary** solution until you can drive to the local tire company for a true fix. But with your health you shouldn't settle for anything other than "a true fix." You wouldn't trust your spare tire to safely deliver you and your loved ones to your many destinations. Why would you accept such an approach for your body? So don't just treat the symptoms when you don't feel your best, look for what is causing the problem. Bottom line, you need to address the cause.

For example, when your favorite team loses a football game, it's easy to blame those last few plays that occur. Sure, a fumble in the final two minutes or the failure to get within field goal range during the final seconds of the game do contribute to the loss, especially if the game is close. The reality is that there are many of these moments that have occurred throughout the game, and a change in any one of them could have turned into a win. Similarly, there are incalculable factors that affect one's health that can bring about premature death: high blood pressure, elevated blood sugar, or decreased immunity. One may look for the reason why the running back didn't have his block or the receiver couldn't get open and attribute these problems to an underlying foundation that the team should have had more practice, or the plays should have been more carefully thought out. Insufficient or imbalanced hormone levels work like the playbook in a football game. When the plays are inadequate or the players don't know them as well as they should, it can cause a myriad of problems on Sunday, and when hormones aren't balanced or aren't sufficient, it can cause a number of diseases. Looking for and treating the **underlying cause** of a problem makes more sense to us, and when one underlying cause can treat a number of symptoms, it makes even more sense! For some reason, we have largely stopped doing this in our modern health care model. If you are suffering from high cholesterol, your doctor will likely prescribe a statin drug (like Lipitor) for you with little or no advice on what the possible causative factors for this condition may be. This is literally akin to the coach blaming the QB exclusively for incomplete passes, and completely ignoring the fact that the offensive line wasn't giving him the time to run the plays.

As we mentioned in the last chapter, it is impossible to talk about the effects of just one hormone on the body. They all work in concert, and the next symptom of testosterone deficiency that we would like to cover is actually more a symptom of estrogen dominance. "Estrogen dominance" is a term coined by the late Dr. John R. Lee to refer to the state when there is a disproportionate amount of estrogen in ratio to progesterone in the body.[21] This balance can be caused by excess estrogen or inadequate progesterone. You may be thinking that this doesn't relate to you, as estrogen and progesterone are the "female hormones," but this balance applies to men just as much as it does to women. Remember, both genders have all of these hormones, but in varying amounts. A man should have significantly less estrogen and progesterone than a woman, but those hormones must still be balanced and fall in a normal physiologic range for men. Even estrogen dominance is connected to testosterone deficiency. Remember when we talked about the relationship of estrogen to testosterone? Testosterone is converted to estrogen by the aromatase enzyme in fat cells. Men with lower

> Salivary reference ranges for men:
> Estradiol – <2.5 pg/ml
> Progesterone – <50 pg/ml
> Prog/E2 ratio – 200–300
> Testosterone – 30.1-142.5 pg/ml
> DHEA – 137-336 pg/ml
>
> - Courtesy of Labrix Clinical Services

levels of testosterone have a decrease in lean body mass, and therefore an increase in fat. Those fat cells are likely to be converting what little testosterone is available into estrogen, which can aggravate an estrogen-dominant environment. Furthermore, when estrogen levels rise, they can trick the hypothalamus to stop signaling to the testes to produce more testosterone and stimulate the liver to produce more SHBG.

Although SHGB binds both testosterone, and estrogen, it has a greater affinity for testosterone, so the total amount of testos-

Healthy: ↑*Testosterone,* ↓*Estrogen,* ↓*SHBG*
Unhealthy: ↓*Testosterone,* ↑*Estrogen,* ↑*SHBG*

terone doesn't change, but the free or bioavailable amount greatly decreases. SHBG rises anyway with age, making this phenomenon even worse. Why is this important? In women, estrogen dominance has been linked to breast and uterine cancer, and studies have shown that the same changes occur in the prostates in men. The prostate actually comes from the same embryologic tissue that the uterus comes from, meaning that in developing male fetuses this tissue becomes a prostate, and in developing female fetuses the tissue becomes a uterus. For this reason, these tissues behave similarly in many ways. Excess amounts of estrogen are known to be associated with prostate gland diseases such as benign prostatic hypertrophy (BPH) and prostate cancer. Prostate problems are among the fastest growing health concerns among men in Western culture.

Prostate cancer accounts for one in three cancers diagnosed in men. The incidence of prostate cancer rises with age, and the majority of men who have prostate cancer are older than 65.[22] Estrogen levels also rise with age, while progesterone and testosterone levels fall. In addition to the excess estrogen produced from fat and regular exposure to xenoestrogens and phytoestrogens (found in pesticides and some food products, respectively) can add to the already-rising estrogen levels and compound the estrogen dominance. While there is a lot of evidence to support the fact that it is actually low testosterone (through this estrogen dominant mechanism) that increases risk of prostate cancer, conventional thought is that high testosterone is what puts you at risk of prostate cancer. There are many things that elevated testosterone levels can increase your risk of, and we will get to that in a minute because it's very important that you understand that only balanced physiological levels of testosterone are safe, but prostate cancer is not caused by testosterone.

In fact, a 2009 study out of Harvard University stated that "studies consistently fail to support the historical idea that T [testosterone] therapy poses an increased risk of prostate cancer or exacerbation of symptoms due to benign prostatic hyperplasia."[23,24] In 1941, Dr. Charles Huggins made the observation that surgical castration appeared to improve the survival of men with prostate cancer compared with men who were not castrated. From this brief study, Dr. Huggins concluded that testosterone was a contributing cause of prostate cancer, and he even won a Nobel Prize for his discovery. Well, prostate cancer is very rare in young men, and increases in incidence as men age and their testosterone levels are declining. Wouldn't you expect to see prostate cancer among younger men who have the highest testosterone levels if, in fact, this was a causative factor? The testes produce more than just testosterone. They are also the glands that produce estrogen and progesterone, so removing them there would correct the estrogen dominance by removing most of the estrogen produced in the male body.[25] Don't worry, you don't need a castration to prevent prostate cancer. Most men just need a little additional progesterone to balance the estrogen levels that are rising in their bodies as they get older.

We often think of prostate problems exclusively with any urinary difficulties, but testosterone also plays a role in bladder capacity and compliance. A recent study out of Turkey followed a number of hypogonadal men on testosterone therapy and found that not only did they report an improvement in sexual function, but the mean maximal bladder capacity increased as well as a decrease in pressure on the detrusor muscle (the muscle that contracts to push urine out of the bladder).[26]

As if it isn't bad enough that the declining testosterone levels are affecting your emotional health (depression) and your physical health (metabolic syndrome, heart disease, and ED), but low testosterone levels are correlated to mental health as well. Testosterone supplementation can enhance cognitive function as well as spatial and verbal memory.[27] Researchers have also discovered that testosterone-deficient rats showed an increased in a beta-amyloid protein which has been implicated in Alzheimer's disease. Sure enough, men with adequate levels of testosterone have demonstrated a decreased incidence of Alzheimer's disease, so these rat studies are showing us the mechanism to a trend that we have already observed.[28] Getting older gracefully requires that you maintain physical, emotional, and mental health. Maintaining healthy physiologic testosterone levels into your "twilight years" will facilitate optimal function of your whole being. Often times the best way to achieve this is through hormone supplementation, but just as there are health concerns with androgen levels that are less than optimal, there are serious dangers to elevated androgen levels. Treatment should be supervised by a physician and lab values monitored closely.

For many people, the idea of testosterone supplementation immediately conjures up images of muscle-bound athletes with horrible tempers due to "doping" or artificial elevation of their androgen levels. In fact, much of what we know about elevated androgen levels comes from studying these athletes who often do irrevocable damage to their bodies in an attempt to win a competition or beat a record. Increased testosterone levels can amplify mood swings and promote aggressive behavior. As mentioned before, there has historically been a lot of concern about the prostate risks associated with testosterone; however, emerging research is showing that enlarged prostates and prostate cancer are more likely attributed to elevated estrogen levels. This doesn't absolve testosterone because, as you should remember, testosterone is converted into estrogen, by the aromatase enzyme in fat tissue, and as testosterone levels rise above physiological levels,

"Lou" is an athletic man with a history of bicycle racing. He came into to the clinic because he had noticed that he was having increasing trouble keeping up with his teammates of the same age, and in general, he was noticing a decrease in energy, motivation, and vitality. Upon testing, we discovered that not only were his testosterone levels significantly declining, but he has a naturally narrow jaw, with a normal-sized tongue that was significantly obstructing his airway. When he slept and tried to repair his muscles after working out, his apnea was preventing his body from getting restorative sleep and was driving his testosterone levels further and further down. Remember, sleep is paramount to your health. **RESTO**RATION of the body starts with the first four letters of the word: REST.

more and more of that testosterone can be converted into estrogen, which can adversely affect the prostate. When the prostate tissue is exposed to elevated estrogen levels without progesterone to balance it, there is an increase risk of BPH and prostate cancer. Testosterone also converts into dihydrotestosterone (DHT). This is done by an enzyme called 5-alpha reductase, which is at its highest concentrations in prostate tissue and hair follicles. DHT has been implicated in male pattern baldness as well as the growth of the prostate. Drugs like Propecia® work to inhibit the enzyme that creates DHT. Because it is an androgen, DHT binds to the same testosterone receptors, but with much greater affinity. Higher than physiologic (normally produced by the body) levels of testosterone can cause more of the hormone to be converted to DHT, and may expedite hair loss and further increase risk of BPH or prostate cancer.

Getting back to the idea of balance, there are many times when we see similar symptoms in the body with too much or too little of a hormone. Just as too little testosterone can cause enlarged breast tissue, the same thing can happen with too much testosterone due to the same mechanism: conversion to estrogen. Most bodybuilders, and even those who haven't used steroids but spend a lot of time in a gym, know that it's important to take "anti-estrogens" to counteract this effect and prevent what is commonly referred to as "gyno" or, as we're told by our bodybuilding friends, the politically incorrect term "bitch tits." As we said before, gynecomastia is not the same thing as simply increased fatty tissue over the chest (pseudogynecomastia). True gynecomastia involves hyperplasia of the mammary glands and can include a transformation of the nipple to look more like a woman's. This tissue doesn't simply go away with weight loss either, and many men have to resort to breast reduction surgery to remove this common symptom of steroid abuse.

A sign of excess testosterone that quickly gets the attention of many men is a decrease in testicle size. This is due to that old feedback mechanism that we discussed in the last chapter. Basically, if the body thinks there's enough androgen hormone in the body, it doesn't see a need to produce any more. When the tissue isn't being used, it shuts down and shrinks up. Remember that testosterone acts locally in the testicle on the Sertoli cells to stimulate sperm production, but when the testicle isn't producing testosterone and begins to shrink, the Sertoli cells shrink as well, reducing or even halting spermatogenesis (sperm production). For this reason, testosterone supplementation is **not** recommended for men who want to remain fertile and, in fact, is even being researched as a possible male contraceptive. The testicle often returns to its normal size and function when testosterone or other androgen supplementation is discontinued, but for

Risks of increased testosterone levels:

- Aggressive behavior
- Gynecomastia
- Testicle shrinking
- Reduced sperm count
- Infertility
- Increased risk of prostate cancer*
- Acne
- Liver tumors or dysfunction
- Altered cholesterol profile
- Thickening of blood (increased hematocrit)
- Central sleep apnea
- Down regulation of androgen receptors

*Note: There are links between excess testosterone and decreased testosterone with prostate cancer risk; maintaining health levels and monitoring any therapy is the key.

men who still want to father a child some day, this is a gamble they may not want to take.

Although appropriate physiologic levels of testosterone have a positive effect on cholesterol, overdosage with testosterone can lower the HDL cholesterol (good cholesterol) and raise the LDL (bad cholesterol), which can adversely affect cardiac health. High levels of testosterone have been shown to increase the hematocrit or red blood cell count as well by stimulating erythropoietin, as we mentioned in the last chapter. The addition of more red blood cells causes the blood to become thicker or more viscous. Think of what the oil in your car looks like when you drain it. I'm sure all of you change your oil on a regular schedule, but imagine if you let it go for a little too long. When you finally pulled the drain plug, you would see thick, dark, sticky clumps of oil that look nothing like the smooth, clean oil that you started with. Just as this old, unchanged oil can cause problems in your engine, thickened blood can cause blockages in your arteries and veins leading to strokes, heart attacks, lung problems, and end organ damage.

It is easy (and important) to monitor your red blood cell count with any testosterone supplementation, and when we get to the chapter on testing, we will suggest you have your liver enzymes checked occasionally as well. Your liver is an amazing organ that functions to manufacture many of the proteins, enzymes, hormones, and immune complexes that are necessary for life, but also to eliminate the toxins and excess endogenous (self-produced) compounds from your body. That being said, there are many medications and substances that can cause such an increase to the load of the liver that it begins to fall behind in its functioning. You are likely aware of the negative effects that alcohol can have on your liver, and most of us have heard about the problems that various medications (even over-the-counter items) can cause. Basically everything that you swallow gets filtered by your liver, and the more we throw at it the harder it has to work and the more likely it is to malfunction. Testosterone supplementation is no different, and oral forms of testosterone have been implicated in many situations of liver toxicity including liver tumors that are both benign and malignant. One symptom of liver dysfunction is jaundice, or the yellowing of skin, eyes, or body fluids due to a buildup of bilirubin in the tissues. Bilirubin is a normal byproduct of the life cycle of red blood cells, but must be processed by the liver. When the liver is overwhelmed with other tasks or not functioning properly, there can be a buildup of many toxins in our system. Bilirubin is just easier to see due to its yellow color. Other symptoms of liver malfunction may include nausea, vomiting, fluid retention, and elevated liver enzymes upon blood testing.

Remember when we were advocating balance? There are many symptoms or problems that can occur due to decreased or elevated testosterone levels, indicating that what is needed is a balance. We covered sleep apnea, a sleep disorder where people stop breathing in their sleep, during the section on low testosterone. Sleep apnea is most commonly caused by an obstruction in the back of the throat, but can also be caused by a modification in the breathing center in the brain. Sleep apnea can contribute to a myriad of health problems including snoring, fatigue, anxiety, high blood pressure, and many others. Non-obstructive sleep apnea, also called central sleep apnea, is not caused by a physical blockage of the airway, and has been linked to testosterone supplementation. It is likely that the testosterone is causing a disruption in the breathing center in the brain, but can cause many of the same disease processes that we see with obstructive sleep apnea.[29] Does this all sound confusing? We just told you how dangerous low testosterone is to your sleep—now we're saying supplementation has been linked to problems as well! Look, all we want you to take away from this is that you should be aware of potential side effects. If you have a history of sleep apnea or your partner notices a worsening of snoring or incidences of stopped breathing, then you should get it checked out.

Though many of the side effects of elevated testosterone levels can be severe, many are often as simple as mimicking the symptoms of puberty—acne, oily skin, and increased body hair have all been reported. These symptoms are far more benign than increased risk of heart attack or liver cancer, but are a nuisance nonetheless. All of these factors need to be taken into account when developing a treatment plan that is safe and effective. Knowing the effects of low and high testosterone levels is key to establishing balance and optimal health in your body as you age. Proper monitoring of lab values and guidance by a trained physician coupled with your own knowledge of the various faces of testosterone will give you the tools you need to optimize your health, balance your hormones, and feel better! In addition to causing the problems we have discussed above, too much testosterone for too long causes the testosterone receptors to shut down. When this occurs, you will see the old symptoms of testosterone insufficiency reappear.

Many men suffering from andropause who were treated and felt better eventually find that they are fatigued again, their brain is cloudy like it used to be, they are gaining weight, and, of course, they find that their libido and ability for erections are sliping away. More is **NOT** always better. Just because a little of something makes you feel good doesn't mean that even more of it will make you feel fantastic, and testosterone is the perfect example. So remember, all things in moderation, not too much, not too little. Like Goldilocks likes her porridge, we want your hormone levels to be just right.

NOTES

1. Langeluddeke, A, *Die Entmannung von Sittlichkeitsverbrecher* (Berlin: de Gruyter, 1963).

2. P. Anderson, *"Low Testosterone Levels Linked With Higher Risk for Depression"* Arch Gen Psychiatry (2008) 65:283–289, http://www.medscape.com/viewarticle/571098?src=mp.

3. Gades, N.M., D.J. Jacobson, M.E. McGree, J.L. St. Sauver, M.M. Lieber, A. Nehra, C.J. Girman, G.G. Klee, S.J. Jacobsen, "The associations between serum sex hormones, erectile function, and sex drive, The Olmsted County Study of Urinary Symptoms and Health Status among Men, *J Sex Med* (2008) Sep; 5(9):2209–20; E-pub (2008) Jul 4.

4. Chamness, S.L., D.D. Ricker, J.K. Crone, C.L. Dembeck, M.P. Maguire, A.A.L. Burnett, T.S. Chang, "The effect of androgen on nitric oxide synthase in the male reproductive tract of the rat," *Fertil Steril* (1995) 63:1101–1107. Zvara, P., R. Sioufi, H.M. Schipper, L.R. Begin, G.B. Brock, "Nitric oxide mediated erectile activity is a testosterone dependent event; a rat erection model," *Int J Impt Res* (1995) 7:209–219.

5. Yassin, A.A., F. Saad, L.J. Gooren, "Metabolic syndrome, testosterone deficiency and erectile dysfunction never come alone," *Andrologia* (2008) Aug, 40(4):259–64.

6. Shabsigh, R., S. Arver, K.S. Chaner, I. Eardley, A. Fabbri, L. Gooren, A. Heufelder, H. Jones, S. Meryn, M. Zitzmann, "The triad of erectile dysfunction, hypogonadism and the metabolic syndrome," Int *J Clin Pract* (2008) May, 62(5):791–8.

7. Kalyani, R.R., and A.A. Dobs, "Androgen deficiency, diabetes, and the metabolic syndrome in men," *Curr Opin Endocrinol Diabetes Obes* (2007) Jun, 14(3):226–34.

8. Gould, D.C., R.S. Kirby, P. Amoroso, "Hypoandrogen-metabolic syndrome: a potentially common and underdiagnosed condition in men," *Int J Clin Pract* (2007) Feb, 61 (2):341–4 17263722 (P, S, E, B, D).

9. Spark, R.F., "Testosterone, diabetes mellitus, and the metabolic syndrome," *Curr Urol Rep*, (2007) Nov, 8(6):467–71.

10. http://diabetes.niddk.nih.gov/dm/pubs/statistics/DM_Statistics.pdf.

11. Phillips, G.B., B.H. Pinkernell, T.Y. Jing, "The association of hypotestosteronemia with coronary artery disease in men," *Arterioscler Thromb* (1994) May, 14(5):701–6.

12. E. C. Tsai, E. J. Boyko, D. L. Leonetti, W. Y. Fujimoto *"Low serum testosterone level as a predictor of increased fixceral fat in Japanese-American men,"* Intern. Journal of Obesity (2000) 24, 485–491.

13. Kapoor, D., E. Goodwin, K.S. Channer, T.H. Jones, "Testosterone replacement therapy improves insulin resistance, glycaemic control, visceral adiposity and hypercholesterolaemia in hypogonadal men with type 2 diabetes," *Eur J Endocrinol* (2006) Jun, 154(6):899–906.

14. *J Clin Endocrinol Metab* (2008) 93:139–146, or http://www.medscape.com/viewarticle/569642.

15. Hak, A.E., J.C. Witterman, F.H. de Jong, et al, "Low levels of endogenous androgens increase the risk of atherosclerosis in elderly men: the Rotterdam study," *J Clin Endocrinol Metab* (2002) Aug, 87(8):3632–9.

16. Tsang, S., S. Wu, J. Liu, T.M. Wong, "Testosterone protects rat hearts against ischaemic insults by enhancing the effects of alpha(1)-adrenoceptor stimulation," *Br J Pharmacol* (2008) Feb, 153(4):693–709; E-pub 2007 Dec 24.

17. Klentze, M. *Testosterone, The Male Hormone Connection: Treating Diabetes and Heart Disease.*

18. R. Klatz, R. Goldman, *"The Anti-Aging Revolution"* Basic Health Publications, 2007.

19. Amory, J.K., "Exogenous testosterone or testosterone with finasteride increases bone mineral density in older men with low serum testosterone," *J Clin Endocrinol Metab* (2004) 89: 503–10.

20. The Endocrine Society press release, accessed online at http://www.endo-society.org/ on June 23, 2008.

21. Lee J.R., and V. Hopkins. *Hormone Balance Made Simple: The Essential How-to Guide to Symptoms, Dosage, Timing and More* (Warner Books Publishing, 2006).

22. National Cancer Institute, "What you need to know about prostate cancer," posted Aug 1, 2005.

23. Morgentaler A., C. Schulman, "Testosterone and prostate safety." *Front Homr Res.* 2009; 37:197–203.

24. *J Natl Cancer Inst*, published online January 29, 2008; 2008;100:158–159, 170–183.

25. Lee, J.R., "Hormone balance for men: What your doctor may not tell you about prostate health and natural hormone supplementation," *Hormones Etc.*, 2003.

26. Karazindiyanoglu, S. and S. Cayan, "The effect of testosterone therapy on lower urinary tract symptoms/bladder and sexual functions in men with symptomatic late-onset hypogonadism," *Aging Male* (2008) Sep, 11(3):146–9.

27. Cherrier, M.M., S. Plymate, S. Mohan, et al, "Relationship between testosterone supplementation and insulin-like growth factor-I levels and cognition in healthy older men," *Psychoneuroendocrinology* (2004) Jan 29(1):65–82.

28. Rosario, E.R., L. Chang, F.Z. Stanczyk, C.J. Pike, "Age-related testosterone depletion and the development of Alzheimer's disease," *JAMA*, Sept 22;292(12):1431–2.

29. Andersen, M.L. and S. Tufik, "The effects of testosterone on sleep and sleep-disordered breathing in men: Its bidirectional interaction with erectile function," *Sleep Med Rev* (2008) Oct 12(5):365–79; E-pub 2008 Jun 5. Barrett-Connor, E., D. Thuy-Tien, K. Stone, S. Litwack Harrison, S. Redline, E. Orwol, "The Association of Testosterone Levels with Overall Sleep Quality, Sleep Architecture, and Sleep-Disordered Breathing," *J Clin Endocrin & Metab*; Vol. 93, No7:2602–2609.

CHAPTER 5

Diseases that Affect Testosterone

By now you should know the role that testosterone plays in the body, and for the most part what happens if we don't have enough of it or if there is too much. We've also told you that testosterone levels naturally drop by about 1 percent per year starting at approximately age 30. It would be nice if that were the whole picture, but unfortunately there are many of us out there with lifestyles and disease processes that are compounding our already declining hormone levels, and many people have it even worse than that as there are several genetic conditions that result in very little or no hormones produced.

A reduction or cessation of testosterone production can be classified as primary, secondary, or tertiary. In primary hypogonadism, it is the testicle that stops producing testosterone for whatever reason. With cases of primary hypogonadism, or testicular failure, the testicles are still receiving the message from the hypothalamus and the pituitary to make the hormone, but there is a problem somewhere in the testicle. This is the most common, and, therefore, it is what we are most concerned with. Remember our analogy about the corporation? Primary hypogonadism is similar to what goes on when there is a labor strike. The instruction to continue producing may still be coming from the CEO and the management team, but there is no product because the employees refuse to or are unable to manufacture the product. With secondary hypogonadism, the testicles continue to function correctly, but the message from the pituitary is disrupted or altered even though the pituitary is getting the correct signal from the hypothalamus. In the corporate setting, if a new procedure was implemented and communicated to the management level, but the message failed to get to the employees, it would be similar to secondary hypogonadism because the break in communication occurred at the management level. Just as it would be in the corporate model, this is not as common as a primary problem like the strike situation. Tertiary hypogonadism occurs when there is a disruption or incorrect signal coming from the hypothalamus to the pituitary, or a lack of message from the CEO. Because they are less common, and therefore less relevant, let's quickly cover secondary and tertiary hypogonadism before we work our way to the more common stuff that will hit a little closer to home.

Kallaman's syndrome is an example of a tertiary hypogonadism. It is a condition that occurs at birth where the hypothalamus doesn't produce the GnRH (gonadotropin-releasing hormone) that tells the pituitary to release the luteinizing hormone (LH) and the follicle stimulating hormone (FSH). The reduction in testosterone and sperm production is usually accompanied by a malfunction of the olfactory nerve, which results in an inability to smell and sometimes an error in the optic nerve, which results in color blindness. This is a syndrome that can happen in both men and women, is usually diagnosed when puberty is delayed, and is treated with hormone supplementation. Kallaman is a serious condition that occurs in approximately 1 in 4,000 births.

Pituitary disorders would all be classified as secondary hypogonadisms and can occur from a variety of causes. Pituitary tumors are more common than Kallaman's syndrome and, in fact, account for approximately 15 percent of all neoplasms[1] (that's a fancy word for new growths) in the brain. Pituitary tumors are often benign (non-cancerous), but can cause the pituitary to increase secretion of one or more of its hormones, or stop secreting hormones altogether. This is why laboratory testing by your physician is important. Often, pituitary tumors or other brain tumors near the pituitary are treated with surgery or radiation, and it is actually the treatment that results in hypogonadism. Inflammatory diseases such as sarcoidosis, tuberculosis, and some fungal infections can involve the hypothalamic-pituitary axis, resulting in a decrease in testosterone production. Viruses such as the HIV virus can attack the hypothalamus, the pituitary, or the testicle itself. It is common for men with HIV or AIDS to concomitantly suffer from significant depletion of testosterone, but it's hard to know exactly what the cause is. The increased stresses on the body from the physical pain, emotional trauma, and social pressures of the disease, combined with the inflammation from opportunistic infections and the taxing effects of all of the medications can all contribute to disruption in hormonal pathways. Whatever the reason for the deficiency, men with HIV and AIDS represent a population that has seen some marked improvement in their symptoms with testosterone supplementation.[2]

If asked what makes you male you may say your penis, your beard, or maybe even your sense of direction, commanding grasp of mechanics, or superior sports knowledge. A normal male has one X chromosome and one Y chromosome, so on the most basic level, it is the Y chromosome that truly defines maleness, since women have two X chromosomes. Klinefelter's syndrome is a genetic condition where the genome of a developing baby has more than one X chromosome but also has a Y chromosome. This confusing genetic signal results in abnormal development of the testicles, low testosterone production, fertility problems, and usually the misfortune of smaller-than-normal testicles. Men with this condition tend to be tall with disproportionately long arms and legs, have small testicles, are likely to develop gynecomastia, and have a predisposition for learning difficulties, but for the most part are normal in appearance. In fact, many men don't even know that they have this genetic abnormality until they seek guidance for infertility problems and look into their genetic code.[3]

Just before birth, the testicles that have developed inside the abdomen of the fetus move down into the scrotum. Though this should occur a month or more before birth, occasionally it hasn't yet happened when the baby is born. This condition, called cryptorchidism, is relatively common among premature infants, affecting approximately 30 percent of them. The condition usually corrects itself within a few years without treatment; however, if it isn't corrected in early childhood, it can lead to a malfunction of the testicle and a reduction in the two major exports of the testicle: testosterone and sperm. A baby born with even one undescended testicle has a higher risk of infertility, testosterone insufficiency, and testicular cancer. The higher temperature inside the body cavity is less than optimal for sperm production and there is a high risk for testicular torsion. For this same reason, it is believed that men that wear briefs instead of boxers may have an increased risk of infertility due to the difference in temperature that can be upwards of four degrees. You may not even know if you had an undescended testicle when you were born; if it corrected itself and didn't cause a problem, then it may have never been mentioned.

So, if you weren't born with one of these genetic or intrauterine abnormalities, you should have normal function of your testicles, right? Well, maybe. There are a lot of situations that can affect your testicles' optimum performance. It's no secret that one of the worst places to strike a man is in his genital region. In fact, most self-defense classes for women advise them to strike the nose and the groin of their attacker since that is where the greatest pain can be inflicted with the smallest amount of force. As you are probably aware, the testicles are very sensitive and trauma in that region causes a great deal of pain. Many of you are probably cringing a bit just recalling the last time you accidently slipped off the bicycle seat onto the crossbar, or were inadvertently struck in the genital area during a playful wrestling match or some other activity. It goes without saying that great care should be made to protect the testicles at all times. For the most part, this is well-understood; nearly all athletes in most sports and at every level wear a cup and a jock strap to protect their manhood. Many athletes would give up their helmet before they'd let go of their cup. The testicles are prone to injury because they have very little to protect them. They are just hanging out there, literally, and can be very vulnerable. We don't need to go into the specific details of the most common types of trauma to the testicle: suffice it to say that it's not a good idea to let anything or anyone kick, hit, whack, punch, squeeze, stab, or bite your testicles. The more this occurs, the greater the risk of your testicles underperforming and that means infertility as well as lowered testosterone levels. If you've had an extreme trauma, such as a testicular rupture or torsion (which occurs when the spermatic cord gets twisted inside the scrotum; it's VERY painful), then you should be even more mindful of your testosterone levels, but even repeated minor strains can cause a problem. One study found increased calcification in extreme mountain bikers compared to nonbikers,[4] and it's believed that the repeated small traumas were what caused them.

Though we don't see it as often anymore due to vaccinations, the mumps virus still occurs occasionally, and, in addition to infecting the salivary glands causing the characteristic lumps in the neck that we often associate with the virus, it can also infect the testicles, causing long-term testicular damage. In 1968, there were 15,209 cases of the mumps virus reported in the United States, but only 1,692 by 1993 (a 99 percent reduction)[5] So mumps is really pretty rare these days, but depending on your age, it's something that may have affected you as a kid and could potentially prevent you from having optimal testicular function.

"George" was in his early thirties when he first read something about testicular cancer and realized he had never really taken a look at his testicles. The next time he was in the shower, he performed a thorough exam and thought he felt something. Of course, he was inclined to think that he was just being paranoid; I mean, what are the odds of finding testicular cancer on your first testicular exam, right? Well, just to be sure, he went to the doctor and discovered he **did** have testicular cancer. That was many years ago, and George is now is doing well. He is a very proud father of three after having one of his testicles removed; however, as he ages he will need to be even more careful and vigilant about watching his hormone levels to maintain optimum health.

Hemochromatosis is an inherited condition where there is too much iron stored in the blood. The iron can become deposited in the organs causing a wide range of problems including heart disease when deposited in the heart, liver cirrhosis and failure when deposited in the liver, diabetes when deposited in the pancreas; and, of course, when the iron becomes deposited in the pituitary, it disrupts endocrine function. Hemochromatosis is relatively common, occurring in approximately 1 in 300 people and more often in men than women. It is often not diagnosed until the patient is 40 or so, and simple blood tests can look at iron storage in the blood, which would indicate if there is a problem.

Cancer is one of those diseases that just about every one of us has come in close contact with. We'd be willing to bet that someone very close to you has had cancer, and you have probably even lost some of your loved ones at the hands of this very diverse disease. Cancer is a very general term used to describe a number of different conditions. Not all cancers are created equally. Some cancers, like pancreatic cancer, have a relatively poor survival rate. Other conditions, such as basal cell carcinoma, a common skin cancer, are technically cancer, yet are frequently treated during an afternoon visit to the doctor and do not have a high likelihood of returning. General cancer screening is a very good idea for everyone, and should be a part of your everyday health care. Chemotherapy or radiation of any kind, for any type of cancer, can dramatically affect your ability to produce testosterone. If you have gone through chemotherapy or radiation therapy for cancer treatment, chances are this matter was discussed with you to some degree. Men who are still at an age where they may want to be fertile often put sperm in a bank in case they don't regain their fertility after treatment. While fertility is most often addressed in these situations, if relevant, the suboptimal testosterone production that results from an irradiated testicle or endocrine system that is damaged by the very toxic chemotherapeutic drugs is often overlooked. It is even more important that you take a look at your hormone levels if your body has been exposed to cancer therapies.

Of course, cancer can affect your testosterone production even more directly. Testicular cancer, for example, is most prevalent in men under the age of 35, a time when most men still believe that they are invincible. Palpating or examining your testicles monthly for any changes (such as hard lumps or painful areas) is a good idea. Women are told to perform monthly breast examinations, and there's no reason why men shouldn't be just as responsible about their health. A few minutes a day could possibly save your life. You can simply do this while you are in the shower; in fact, the soap makes it easy to slide your fingers around the testicles and feel throughout the scrotum, plus the warm water makes the scrotum relaxed. A healthy testicle should feel somewhat like a peeled hardboiled egg, with a lump (called the epididymis) on top and a cord that extends up from that into your abdominal wall. You should feel for any changes, anything you notice in one side and not the other, and especially for any hard, immobile objects. Testicular cancer has one of the highest cure rates of all cancers, so catching it early is the key. Lance Armstrong had testicular cancer, was treated for it, and went on to win more Tour de France races than anyone in history!

Ok, so you don't have Klinefelter's or Kallaman's syndrome. You've never had cancer or been treated with chemotherapy drugs. No doctor has ever told you that you had a problem with your iron storage. You're pretty sure you never had mumps, and you've always been very careful about protecting your testicles. You should be good, right? Well, not necessarily. While these are well-documented causes of hypogonadism, for most people the explanation isn't quite so simple. For most of us, the impact of medications (prescribed, over-the-counter, and recreational), alcohol use, stress, and aging (or a combination of these factors) all lead to a diminishing testosterone level. Sometimes many of the diseases that are caused by low testosterone turn out to be further causes of even lower testosterone, creating a self-perpetuating cycle.

In the last chapter, we discussed how low testosterone levels cause depression, but it seems that the opposite is also true. This may be a chicken-and-egg scenario, but a team of doctors in Germany found that sex hormones are secreted at different rates in men who are severely depressed than in men who are not. An exact mechanism for this hasn't yet been clarified, but the team of doctors also found a 68-percent-higher cortisol concentration in the men with depression, and cortisol is known to have an inverse relationship with testosterone.[6] It may be worth noting that the study subjects were only those who exhibited extremely severe depression, and mildly depressed individuals were ruled out. It's possible that the severe depression causes such a stress response that the high cortisol (a stress hormone) is the reason for the low testosterone, or they may be coincidental. They did test the concentrations of LH and FSH (the pituitary hormones that stimulate the testicles to make testosterone and sperm) and found them to be similar to the control group overall; however, LH is released in surges and this seemed to occur less often in the depressed group than in the non-depressed men.

Another chicken-and-egg situation is that of elevated cholesterol and impaired glucose metabolism (or metabolic syndrome). Remember that metabolic syndrome is probably one of the most important effects of low testosterone because it is the clogged arteries and heart attacks that will kill you. Low libido is an important symptom to treat because sex is an important part (or should be an important part) of a healthy relationship and a healthy life, but it won't literally kill you if you aren't in the mood. Let's explain quickly what happens in a heart attack. Your heart is a large muscle that pumps blood through the miles and miles of arteries, capillaries, and veins in your body. When your heart beats, half of it sends blood through your lungs to become oxygenated, and the other half receives the oxygenated blood from your lungs and sends it out into the body to deliver the oxygen to the tissues. This much you probably know. (We realize this is Biology 101, especially if you have a background in science or even took an anatomy and physiology class sometime in college, but since there are many people who either haven't had anyone explain fundamental biology or don't remember every detail they learned in college 20 or 30 years ago, bear with us for just a minute.) Back to the heart. It's a powerful muscle that needs quite a bit of oxygen just for itself. Though it weighs in at an average of only 10 ounces, it beats an average of 72 times per minute, meaning that it contracts 103,680 times per day and pumps blood through 60,000 miles of blood vessels to reach the 75 trillion cells that comprise the body. When the oxygenated blood returns from the lungs, a small amount of it is shunted into a blood supply that goes specifically to the heart tissue via the coronary arteries, and not into the interior cavity of the heart that pumps the blood. (Like when you bake cookies, a little taste for the cook and the rest to the oven.)

When you have elevated cholesterol, too much glucose and high triglycerides (all part of the metabolic syndrome picture) in your blood can cause damage inside the small blood vessels. This can happen anywhere along the 60,000 miles of blood vessels in the body, but there are few places where it's as important as the heart tissue. When the damage occurs inside an artery, our body tries to repair it just like it repairs a tear in our skin, with a little scab or clot. Sometimes a clot can become so big that it completely blocks an artery or breaks loose and travels to a smaller artery where it can become lodged and prevent the tissue from getting the blood and oxygen that it needs to function. When this occurs in the heart,it is called a heart attack. If the same process occurs in the brain, it results in a stroke. If the problem is corrected quickly enough, the tissue may live, but if any tissue in the body goes without oxygen for too long it will die. Imagine what it feels like to block off the blood to the tip of your finger. Have you ever put a rubber band around your finger or carried a plastic grocery sack that was heavy and all of the pressure was on a small part of your finger? First you get an intense cramping pain, and eventually your fingertip, like your heart muscle or brain tissue, will die without oxygen. Just as lack of oxygen due to blocked arteries can cause a heart attack or a stroke, or your fingertip to die, blocked arteries can also prevent blood flow to the testicle which causes a decrease in testosterone production.

Surprisingly, there are mixed reviews in the literature about smoking and hypogonadism. Some studies find that cigarettes raise testosterone levels and some find that it lowers them, but scientific studies are in agreement that smoking is NOT good for your cardiovascular health.[7] If you are a smoker, you probably don't want to hear another couple of doctors advising you to quit. You probably know the negative effects that each cigarette has on your body and have your reasons for continuing to smoke. Cigarettes contribute to atherosclerosis, which restricts blood flow significantly to the testes and the penis and plays a large role in erectile dysfunction as well as decreased testosterone levels. Of course, there are a number of reasons that cigarettes are bad for you: the thousands of chemicals that add to your liver burden, the buildup of tar and smoke in your lungs, the chronic inflammation in your bronchial passages, the barrage of carcinogens your body is exposed to . . . the list goes on and on. So here's one more reason to quit if you can't do it for any other reason: do it for your testicles!

Depending on where you live in the country and what generation you grew up in, you may or may not smoke marijuana. Or maybe you did when you were younger, but gave it up as you became more mature or had more adult responsibilities. Well, if you haven't given it up yet, it's time to consider it as there is some evidence to support the fact that some of the chemicals found in marijuana disrupt the formation of androgen hormones and there are some constituents of the plant that show estrogen-like activity.[8] While for many of you this information isn't relevant, you might be surprised at how many people smoke marijuana on a regular basis, or did smoke it for a significant portion of their lives despite the fact that it remains illegal. A 2004 study in the *Journal of the American Medical Association* estimated that marijuana use has remained at a stable 4% over the last decade.[9] And that number is, of course, only reflective of the people who report it: there are likely many others who choose to maintain their privacy.

One drug that is legal and is even more widely used than marijuana is alcohol. Chances are pretty good that you consume alcohol at least on an occasional, social basis. Now keep in mind that moderation is the key to all things, so you don't need to take this information so seriously that you refuse to have an occasional beer if you are so inclined. That's not the intention here. We just want you to know that when you consume a six-pack several nights a week, you can be dramatically affecting your testosterone levels. It has long been understood that testosterone levels are affected adversely by alcohol use; however, a study in 2003 indicated that there may be a short-term increase in testosterone levels with alcohol use, but an overall suppression of production with chronic use.[10] This rise in testosterone initially may be responsible for the typical "bar fight" scenario where a usually calm man can become enraged and aggressive because he is drunk. Or it may simply be that alcohol, which is a known depressant, is preventing your rational mind from being in control of your normal underlying primal impulses. It seems that the mechanism for the lowered testosterone production occurs at all three levels of production (hypothalamic, pituitary, and gonadal). With chronic alcohol abuse, not only does the testosterone level decrease, but also the LH and GnRH levels.[11] In addition, there is evidence to support the theory that alcohol reduces the number of LH receptors in the testes, which then results in less testosterone.[12] The bottom line here is that there have been many studies for many years that equate excessive alcohol use with decreased testosterone levels, and this appears to happen via several mechanisms.[13] What is excessive, you ask? Well, the definition of alcoholism is somewhat subjective and usually comes down to something like this: the continuing use of alcohol despite the health or social problems it may cause. You may not consider yourself to be an "alcoholic" and yet you may certainly be consuming enough alcohol to affect your endocrine system. Furthermore, if the alcohol you are consuming is affecting your health and you continue to drink despite this fact, it does to some degree define you as an alcoholic. The purpose of this book is not to define alcoholism for you, or advise you what safe and healthy amounts of alcohol are. Simply take a look at your consumption. If it's a significant part of your life, chances are it's playing a significant role in suppressing your testosterone production.

There are several theories about the total stress that we are subjected to due to an over-stimulated environment. Think about it, and see how close this fits to your life. You are surfing the Internet, navigating through a new pop-up ad with each page, the TV is on, and you are casually following the episode of *Law and Order* while you are chatting on the phone with your brother. Or maybe you are driving in traffic while listening to the radio, the kids screaming in the backseat and you're talking on your Bluetooth. Our bodies have to process all information that we encounter, and we live in a world where we are constantly bombarded with new input and this can take a toll on our adrenal system, which in turn can affect the rest of the endocrine system, including your sex hormones and your blood sugar regulation.

So far we've covered a couple of congenital abnormalities as well as some lifestyle choices that are responsible for less-than-optimal testosterone levels. What if these situations don't apply to you at all? You don't drink or smoke, you exercise regularly, you eat a relatively healthy diet, yet you are still having many of the symptoms of low androgens that you saw listed back in chapters 1 and 4. Here's something that affects all of us: **stress**. Stress can be defined as any outside force or event that has an effect on our body or our mind. The stressor may be physical, emotional, or mental and its effects can be very far-reaching. In our society, we generally talk about stress as a negative, but stressors can be good things as well as bad. Stress can come from a new relationship, or moving to a new home, or certainly from having a new baby or new puppy in the house. All of these events would generally be thought of as positive; however, they are all outside forces that are affecting us. When our bodies perceive a stressor, it causes a stress response. The varying degree of stress perceived will vary the stress response.

You have probably experienced what it feels like to have an acute stress response. Imagine yourself driving on an icy road. You have had plenty of experience driving in the snow and are relatively relaxed just driving along listening to your favorite CD. The light a block away turns red and you gently press on the breaks with plenty of time to slow to a stop, but the car starts to slide. You must be on some black ice because you completely lose control of the car. You are now sliding toward the intersection, the car starts to turn sideways, and you realize there is no way you are going to be able to stop in time to avoid sliding through the light. You brace yourself for the impact while still scrambling to steer the car and regain control. Eventually you slide to a stop and realize that you are no longer moving; you didn't run into anything, and the cars around you were all able to stop to avoid hitting you. You quickly move your car out of the intersection and pull over into a parking lot a few blocks down to recover. You are out of danger now, but your heart is still racing, your breath is quick, and you feel shaky all over. You take a couple of big breaths to try to relax and regain your composure before continuing on your trip.

There are several reactions that occur in your body during a stress response like this. Your body immediately releases epinephrine, and this is responsible for the initial response that you have during those first few minutes. At the same time though, the good old hypothalamus releases a hormone called corticotrophin releasing hormone (CRH) that then causes the pituitary to release adrenocorticotropic hormone (ACTH). The ACTH acts on the adrenal glands, two glands located on top of your kidneys that produce cortisol and DHEA. Epinephrine rises quickly at the start of a stress response, but then falls quickly as well. Cortisol is just as important, but is a slower response, rising gradually and then sticking around longer. Cortisol's role is to help you sustain a stress reaction beyond the first minute or two, and DHEA helps to control your emotions and provide you with the mental clarity to guide you through the crisis.

Now, you probably aren't sliding around on the ice every day, but our bodies have a similar response to stressors that you probably experience fairly often: stress from our relationships, our jobs, our busy schedules where we are rushing around from one place to another; stress from traffic or from paying our bills. Sound familiar? These are all chronic stressors that we subject our bodies to every day. You may not get the same noticeable response as you did in the near car accident where your heart pounds, your palms get sweaty, and you feel jittery and shaky, but your cortisol production is stimulated, and then stimulated again before it has a chance to normalize. The end result is that many of us live in a state where we are constantly bathed in cortisol. This has several adverse effects, including increasing your blood sugar levels (which creates metabolic syndrome), preferentially storing fat in your abdomen, and suppressing your testosterone and sperm production. When your body is preparing itself for a crisis, it shuts down the functions that aren't immediately needed. Cortisol is our fight-or-flight hormone and is typically elevated when our bodies perceive danger. Our bodies are "designed" to react to an acute stressor so that we can protect ourselves. The stress response causes body functions that are necessary to remove us from danger to become active, while "temporarily" shutting down body functions that aren't beneficial to getting us out of trouble.

For example, an acute stress response, or the reaction you would have to an immediate stressor such as a car accident, is not much different from the reaction that a cat would have when being chased by the neighbor's dog. The heart rate goes up to provide plenty of blood to tissues that need it, the blood is shunted preferentially to the large muscles for running or climbing out of danger, the breath quickens to keep up with the increased oxygen demand, and the eyes dilate so that they can bring in as much information as possible. The stomach and intestines's blood supply is diminished, as it's not important to be digesting food while you are immediately threatened. (You can get to that later when you are safe and calm. (Blood supply to the gonads can also be shunted elsewhere because, while procreation is important for propagation of the species, it's not going to help the cat get over the fence away from the dog, nor is it going to help you stop that car from sliding on the ice. Since our bodies were created much like other mammals, including the cat, we should be able to respond to a stressful event and then recover, allowing our cortisol levels to return to normal. When we have one stressful event after another, or live in a constant state of stress without the break or opportunity to recover completely, the adrenal glands can become worn out and stop making cortisol altogether. This is a very complex system and reaction on which there have been many good books written, but for our purposes, we just want you to understand two things: First, it's important to test your cortisol levels because, secondly, the endocrine system is interconnected and changes in one hormone can greatly affect the levels of other hormones.

In fact, stress may be the primary factor in altered hormone levels for all of us. Erin Lommen, ND, and Jay Mead, MD, founders of Labrix Clinical Services and clinicians with combined experience of over 30 years, have found that adrenal dysfunction almost always accompanies imbalances in sex hormones. Furthermore, they have noticed a trend amongst the tens of thousands of lab tests they have seen that more and more people are suffering from adrenal burnout, and it's occurring in relatively young populations. The conventional medical world tends to ignore adrenal problems until the adrenal glands literally stop producing cortisol altogether. Complete absence of cortisol production is called Addison's disease and is often an autoimmune disease, meaning that it's caused when your immune system accidentally attacks a part of your body that it shouldn't, in this case, your adrenal glands.

As you can imagine, there is a lot of grey area between a normal functioning adrenal system and the Addison's-like picture where there is less than a trace of cortisol when tested. We started out talking about an acute stress response where the cortisol levels would be elevated; eventually though, the overuse of the system causes the adrenal glands to be unable to keep up and they slip into what we call adrenal fatigue and eventually adrenal failure. Evaluating adrenal function is an important part of the workup for andropause as cortisol is known to affect testosterone levels. High levels of cortisol have been shown to inhibit the enzyme that is involved in the biosynthesis of testosterone as well as induce apoptosis (programmed cell death) in Leydig cells[14] which results in a reduced number of Leydig cells, which as you'll remember, are the cells in the testes that produce testosterone. Some of this should be ringing bells for you, but of course, the picture is never completely simple and there are factors other than cortisol and testosterone that are impacting your hormone picture.

We have mentioned several times the important role of estrogen for men's health as well as women's. Remember that estrogen levels rise as testosterone levels fall, partly due to the role of SHBG preferentially binding to testosterone and partly due to the increased conversion of testosterone to estrogen by the aromatase enzyme found in adipose (fat) cells. As your testosterone levels decline, your lean body mass decreases and your body composition migrates toward a greater percentage of fat tissue. This increase in fat tissue exacerbates the conversion to estrogen, causing a spiral effect that is difficult to get ahold of. Studies have even shown that there is a correlation between the degree of obesity and estrogen levels.[15] Another big factor that contributes to estrogen dominance for both genders is the presence of estrogen-like compounds and other endocrine disruptors in the environment. These compounds vary from synthetic chemicals that may be found in plastics, solvents, pesticides, pharmaceuticals, product additives, cosmetics, birth control pills, and insecticides to substances found in nature such as molds, clover, soy, legumes, and some fruits and vegetables. Many of these compounds look like estrogens, and are referred to as phytoestrogens when they come from plants or xenoestrogens when they come from somewhere else (*xeno* simply means strange). We have known about the "estrogen-like" effects of many plants for a long time and sometimes use them as medicines for that very reason. In men, these compounds can greatly contribute to the proliferation of prostate tissues and further tip the scales of hormone balance.[16]

Compounding the imbalance, most of the cows raised in this country are fed with hormones to increase the rate of growth of the animals so that the dairy and beef industries can increase profits. We are now discovering through more sensitive testing methods that a more significant amount of those hormones remains in the meat and dairy products and is ingested by the consumer than was originally thought. There are varying opinions about what this all means and much of the research on the effects has yet to be done; however, these chemicals and food additives have been implicated in the increased incidence of many cancers (including prostate, breast, and uterine), a number of birth defects including malformation of sex organs,[17] as well as the increasingly early onset of puberty among our children. The Center for Disease Control (CDC) identified 148 potentially toxic chemicals that we are exposed to—and that can have an effect on our health—in the *Third National Report on Human Exposure to Environmental Chemicals*.[18] Though we most often hear about the estrogen-like effects of endocrine-disrupting compounds, there are several chemicals that affect androgen receptors as well. In fact, one of the breakdown products of DDT (an insecticide that was banned for use in the United States in 1972, but continues to be used in many parts of the world) is known to block androgen (testosterone) receptors.[19] You may be thinking that if this compound was banned over 30 years ago, then it shouldn't be a problem, but it's still legal to manufacture it in the United States and sell it to other countries, some of whom we purchase food from and feed to our children and ourselves.

Another source of endocrine-disrupting chemicals are the pharmaceutical drugs that have become so much a part of our society. Actually, chances are slim that most of you reading aren't taking at least one pharmaceutical every day, and, depending on your age, that number could be five or even ten. The average number of retail prescriptions per capita increased from 7.9 in 1994 to 12.3 in 2005 according to the Henry J. Kaiser foundation survey and report in 2006.[20] These drugs are ubiquitous and are finding their way into our water supply, so that even those people who aren't taking any medications are likely affected by the residual buildup in the environment. An ongoing USGS investigation of Lake Mead has discovered detectable amounts of over 13 pharmaceutical drugs as well as other chemicals that are affecting the reproduction and endocrine systems of the fish.[21] This article and study hasn't proven that the water has the same effects on humans, but it still makes you think twice about your sources of food and water.

Chances are pretty good that one or more of the situations described in this chapter apply to you. Very few of us grow all of our own food or are even able to eat exclusively organically grown fruits and vegetables and local, grass-fed, hormone-free animals. Only a minute percentage of people in America are taught to effectively deal with their stress and most all of us are exposed to chemicals on a regular basis, even when we are careful.[22] So, in addition to those birthdays that just keep ticking by, you are likely experiencing a number of additional influences that are adversely affecting your hormone levels.

NOTES

1. M. H. Beers, R. Berkow, *The Merck Manual, Seventeenth Edition*, John Wiley & Sons, 1999, p. 1443.

2. Hengge, U.R., "Testosterone replacement for hypogonadism: clinical findings and best practices," *AIDS Read* (2003) Dec 13(12 Suppl):S15–21.

3. *Merck Manual, Seventeenth Edition*, p. 2239.

4. Frauscher, F., A. Klauser, A. Stenzl, G. Helweg, B. Amort, D. zur Nedden, "US findings in the scrotums of extreme mountain bikers," *Radiology* (2001) May;219(2):427–31.

5. http://www.cdc.gov/mmwR/preview/mmwrhtml/00038546.htm.

6. "Depression May Lower Your Sex Hormones," *ScienceDaily* (May 26, 1999).

7. English, K.M., P.J. Pugh, H. Parry, N.E. Scutt, K.S. Channer, T.H. Jones, "Effect of cigarette smoking on levels of bioavailable testosterone in healthy men," *Clinical Science* (2001) 100, 661–665 (printed in Great Britain).

8. Watanabe, K., E. Motoyo, N. Matsuzawa, T. Funahashi, T. Kimura, T. Matsunaga, K. Arizono, I. Yamamoto, "Marijuana extracts possess the effects like the endocrine disruptime chemicals," *Toxicology* (2005) Jan 31;206(3):471–8.

9. Compton, W.M., Grant, B.F., Colliver, J.D., Glantz, M.D., Stinson, F.S., "Prevalence of marijuana use disorders in the United States," *JAMA*, 2004;291:2114–2121.

10. *Alcoholism: Clinical & Experimental Research*, January 2003 Wiley-Blackwell.

11. Cicero, T.J., "Alcohol-induced deficits in the hypothalamic-pituitary-luteinizing hormone axis in the male," *Alcoholism: Clinical and Experimental Research*," 6:207–215, 1982.

Chiao, Y.B., and D.H. van Thiel, "Biochemical mechanisms that contribute to alcohol-induced hypogonadism in the male," *Alcoholism: Clinical and Experimental Research* 7(2):13 1–134, 1983.

12. Bhalla, V.K., V.P. Rajan, M.E. Newman, "Alcohol-induced luteinizing hormone receptor deficiency at the testicular level," *Alcohol Clin Exp Res* (1983) Spring;7(2):153–62.

13. Ellingboe, J., "Acute effects of ethanol on sex hormones in non-alcoholic men and women," *Alcohol Alcohol Suppl* (1987) 1:109–116.

14. Hardy, M.P., H.B. Gao, Q. Dong, R. Ge, Q. Wang, W.R. Chai, X. Feng, C. Sottas, "Stress hormone and male reproductive function," *Cell Tissue Res* (2005) Oct;322(1):147–53; E-pub 2005 Nov 3.

Gao, H.B., H. Tong, Y.Q. Hu, Q.S. Guo, R. Ge, M.P. Hardy, "Glucocorticoid induces apoptosis in rat leydig cells," *Endocrinology* (2002) Jan;143(1):130–8.

15. Soygur, T., B. Kupeli, K. Aydos, S. Kupeli, N. Arikan, Y.Z. Muftuoglu. "Effect of obesity on prostatic hyperplasia: its relation to sex steroid levels," *Int Urol Nephrol* (1996) 28:55–59.

16. Cheek, A.O., P.M. Vonier, E. Oberdorster, B.C. Burow, J.A. McLachlan. "Environmental signaling: a biological context for endocrine disruption," *Environ Health Perspect* (1998) Feb;106 suppl 1:5–10.

17. Imajima, T., T. Shono, O. Zakaria, S. Suia, "Prenatal phthalate causes cryptochidism postnatally by inducing transabdominal ascent of the tests in fetal rats." *Journal of Pediac Surgery.* 1997 Janj 32(1):18–21.

18. *Third National Report on Human Exposure to Environmental Chemicals*, Centers for Disease Control and Prevention (2005) Atlanta, GA.

19. Kelse, W.R., C.R. Stone, S.C. Laws, E.L. Gray, J.A. Kemppainen, E.M. Wilson, "Persistent DDT Metabolite p,p'-DDE is a Potent Androgen Receptor Antagonist," *Nature* 1995 Jun 15; 375(6532):581–5.

20. http://www.kff.org/rxdrugs/upload/3057–05.pdf.

21. http://pubs.usgs.gov/fs/2006/3131/.

22. Zitzmann, M., *Mechanisms of disease: pharmacogenetics of testosterone therapy in hypogonadal men. Nat Cion Proct Urol.* 2007 Mar; 4(3):161–6.

CHAPTER 6

Aging and Testosterone

By now, you should be well informed of the fact that testosterone levels decline with age since we've probably told you that at least three times a chapter for the first half of this book. What we haven't mentioned yet is growth hormone. Most of you have likely heard of human growth hormone (or HGH) as it's often discussed in the media in relation to sports enhancement and anti-aging treatments. If we are to write a companion to this book, it would likely be about HGH because its effects are as nuanced and varied as those of testosterone. In fact, there are many parallels we could draw between growth hormone and testosterone: they both start declining in the third or fourth decade and fall at a relatively steady rate, and both involve pathways in the body that begin with the hypothalamic-pituitary axis. Actually, HGH is the most abundant hormone produced by the pituitary gland! Both testosterone and HGH are adversely affected by unhealthy lifestyles, and they are both supplemented legally and illegally to enhance performance. As you may guess from the name, growth hormone is responsible for building up tissues including muscle and bone. To simplify, an excess of growth hormone causes gigantism and a deficiency causes a form of dwarfism. Growth hormone is given to dairy cows and cattle being ranched for their meat to increase their growth. Many athletes supplement HGH to give them a competitive edge, make them bigger and stronger, and less prone to injury. HGH is also popular in anti-aging circles and has been called the "fountain of youth."[1] In 1990, a clinical trial of HGH with elderly men found that "the effects of six months of human growth hormone on lean body mass and adipose-tissue mass were (inversely) equivalent in magnitude to the changes incurred during 10 to 20 years of aging."[2] Despite many studies that show remarkable results with HGH treatment, it still remains a somewhat controversial topic. Growth hormone is more difficult to supplement than testosterone and is also significantly more expensive.

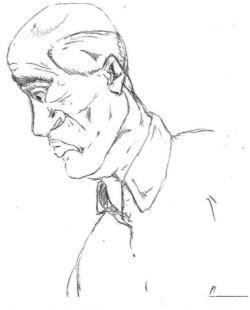

Figure 6.1 Declining testosterone levels leave
many men feeling depressed and with low energy.

We'll save the debate on what to do about declining HGH levels for another
day, but it's important to recognize that growth hormone levels do decline as
we age and mirror testosterone levels in that regard. We keep telling you this
and of course you could just believe us because we have a couple of letters after
our names that give us some credibility, but if you are anything like we are, you
probably want to know more than just the fact that it happens. You want to know
why. "Why?" is almost always a good question to ask. In fact, when it comes to
your health, we recommend you ask as many questions as you can. You're only
given one body and no one can be responsible for it but you. There are a lot
of resources available to you, and you should certainly use them. If you aren't
feeling your best, then you should seek the council of your medical doctor, your
therapist, your naturopathic physician, your nutritionist, your chiropractor, your
friends, and of course the Internet; but ultimately, don't let the FDA, the AMA,
the pharmaceutical industry, or the insurance company tell you what is or is not
acceptable to your health.

Back to the big question: Why? So why do hormone levels change as we age?
As with most "why" questions, the answer isn't entirely simple. We've covered
many of the ways that various diseases and outside influences affect testosterone
and other hormones, and of course the effects of these mechanisms are often
difficult to differentiate from the effects of aging. It's really all tied together,
and we even treat aging as a disease all on its own! Of course, aging is not
an official diagnosis according to the International Classification of Diseases,
but that doesn't mean that we can't treat and prevent many of the processes
of aging. There are a number of theories on aging and with each comes some

new insight on how best to combat this process to extend the quality of our lives, not just the quantity of years we are alive. Each of these theories is a different way of thinking about aging; each offers a different perspective and different avenue to treat aging and disease, and many of these processes exist simultaneously.

WEAR AND TEAR THEORY OF AGING

We can agree that a good general definition for aging would be the accumulation of changes in an organism or object over time. One theory of aging simply states that we age as a consequence of the "wear and tear" we expose our bodies to. Do the math: is the wear and tear you put on your

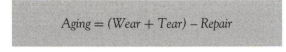

$$Aging = (Wear + Tear) - Repair$$

body exceeding your repair? If so, it is time to do something about it. This is certainly an idea that you are probably familiar with. Have you ever referred to someone as having a "rough life" or maybe as having "a lot of miles under their belt," someone in whom you can literally see the wear and tear they have put on their bodies? Picture the man you pass on the way to work every day who is asking for change on the side of the highway. His skin is leathery from all of the sun, the wrinkles in his face are deep, and when he walks his body is stiff. Someone like this has had more wear and tear on his body than your average individual. As the equation states, it's not just the wear and tear, but also the ability to repair. This is where sleep comes in as such an important part of your overall health. Sleep is your body's opportunity to put all of its energy into repairing the erosion of the day.

Dr. August Weismann, a biologist in Germany, introduced the "wear and tear" theory in 1882. The theory states that the body is damaged and worn down by the toxins in our environment, and this damage occurs on a cellular level. Of course our bodies experience "normal" wear and tear in the process of our daily activities, and eventually our organs will start to falter due to these effects, but we accelerate this process by overusing and abusing our bodies. We lose the ability to repair ourselves from damage caused by environmental toxins, stress, pathogenic organisms, too many shots of tequila, not enough sleep, etc. It is important to remember that the average adult human is comprised of a total of 75 trillion cells, 100 billion brain cells, 60,000 miles of blood vessels, and a heart that weighs a mere 10 ounces yet pumps 100,000 times a day on average. That leaves a lot to repair! Your body has an amazing ability to restore itself, and if given the correct nourishment and care, it can give you the ride of a lifetime, literally. We see patients all the time in our practices that are well into their eighties and nineties and are still devouring life. Picture your car. It has an average lifespan of approximately 145,000 miles according to the U.S. Department of Transportation. But that's average; you know that if you change the oil and filters regularly, put high quality gasoline in it, and drive it relatively conservatively, it could go for twice as many miles. On the other hand, if you let your teenage son or daughter drive it, run it when it's missing a quart or two of oil, or drive in extreme conditions, you'll start having problems way before you would otherwise expect. The average life expectancy of a NASCAR vehicle is approximately 10 races, and the race distances vary from 250–500 miles. So, the cars run approximately 35,000 miles in their lifetime. Only 35,000 miles, and the engines are still practically rebuilt after each race because the extremely demanding conditions cause the systems to breakdown so much sooner than an average car. Our bodies aren't all that different from our cars. If we take good care of them, don't fill them with partially hydrogenated oils, cigarette smoke, and alcohol, and give them the proper rest and relaxation time, then they are likely to run a lot longer than we would otherwise expect—still, how many men do you know who will pay an extra 30 cents per gallon for premium gasoline for their favorite set of wheels, yet fuel their own bodies with dollar menu items from the local burger joint?

CROSS-LINKAGE THEORY OF AGING

Another theory states that aging is due to cross-linkage of proteins causing our cells and tissues to become more rigid and less elastic. Dr. Johan Bjorksten of Finland, a PhD in protein chemistry, developed the Cross-Linkage Theory of Aging in 1942 based on his research with hectograph films (gelatinous films used in early printing processes) that would become hardened and less flexible over time. He found this process to be similar to the changes that occur in human skin and went on to spend much of his life studying cross-linking of proteins and how to delay their formation or dissolve those that had been formed. Dr. Bjorksten theorized that by controlling the cross-linking he could prevent a number of age-related diseases such as osteoporosis, atherosclerosis, cancer, Alzheimer's disease, and endocrine dysfunction. The tanning of leather is a great example of the effects of cross-linking proteins. The soft, supple animal hide becomes rigid, tough, and more durable as the collagen fibers form cross-linking bonds when under the influence of chemicals and heat, reinforcing the structure of the collagen matrix. When these cross-linkages form between bioactive protein molecules, it can render those molecules inactive and disrupt metabolic pathways, inhibit the transfer of genetic information, and cause large inert molecules to accumulate in the cellular matrix that are unable to be transported through the membrane to be removed from the cell.

There is clear and decisive evidence that cross-linking and a process called glycation is accelerated with increased intake of sugar, carbohydrates, and high-glycemic index foods. Glycation is the process of a sugar molecule attaching to a protein or lipid molecule. Sometimes this occurs in the presence of an enzyme in various metabolic pathways and is called glycosylation, but if it just randomly occurs, then it's called simply glycation. During the period of 1970 to 1996, the intake of added sugars in the diet primarily in the form of soft drinks, snacks, desserts, and sweetened juice rose by 23 percent.[3] In addition to the increased amount of sugar, there has been a significant change in the type of sugar that we ingest. Read the labels. Most of our foods are now sweetened with high fructose corn syrup (HFCS) instead of sugar. HFCS is also added to many foods as a preservative, and you may be surprised to find that it's used in many foods that aren't even sweet! Table sugar is made from one molecule of fructose and one molecule of sucrose.

Conditions related to cross-linking:

- Diabetes
- Cognitive decline
- Cancer: including colon, breast, and endometrial
- Depression
- Heart disease
- Hypertension (high blood pressure)
- Increased weight gain
- Cataracts

High fructose corn syrup is commonly 90 percent fructose and 10 percent sucrose. Why is this significant? Because fructose has been found to be ten times as active in glycating proteins as sucrose.[4] This trend toward increased carbohydrate intake overall, coupled with the change in the types of sugars we are ingesting, has accelerated cross-linkage and glycation as well as conditions such as diabetes, obesity, and cardiovascular disease. In 2005, there were 1.5 million individuals diagnosed with diabetes, and there are at least 20 million diabetics in the United States currently. Many individuals may be walking around with diabetes and not even know it yet. It is also estimated that some 50 million Americans suffer from the pre-diabetic state of metabolic syndrome. So, does the aging cause metabolic syndrome or the other way around? It's all in how you look at it. Blood sugar imbalances and insulin resistance will certainly accelerate premature biological aging.

Take a look at the list of conditions associated with cross-linking; it's like looking at the *Who's Who* of top killers of today's society. But how does all of this affect testosterone levels? The cross-linking of proteins to each other or proteins to sugars leads to the formation of large waste products in the cells called advanced glycosylation end products (AGEs). These AGEs are bulky, inactive proteins that disrupt normal cell processes including the production of testosterone and the ability for existing testosterone to effectively bind to receptors and stimulate the desired reaction. AGEs collect in the cells and can decrease elasticity and fluidity in cells throughout the body. Think of each one of your cell membranes turning into leather. You may want to be wearing thick leather if you're ever involved in a motorcycle accident, but you certainly don't want your cells to be wearing little leather jackets. Our body processes depend on open and effective communication between our cells. Although AGEs primarily cause problems and disease in our system, we have used this knowledge to develop a laboratory test that helps us evaluate long-term blood sugar control in diabetics. The test is called a hemoglobin A1C, and determines the percentage of hemoglobin (a protein in red blood cells that carries oxygen) that is bound to a sugar molecule. Since red blood cells have a lifespan of approximately 120 days, we can tell what an approximate average blood sugar level has been over the past 3 months.

FREE-RADICAL THEORY OF AGING

The free-radical theory of aging was developed in 1956 at the University of Nebraska by Denham Harman, MD, and asserts that our cells are exposed to free radicals and that the damage from these interactions accumulates in our cells over time. In some ways, this theory is similar to the cross-linking theory as they both describe how we end up with an accumulation of debris in our cells that prohibits proper cellular function. A free radical is a molecule that has an unpaired electron giving it a negative charge. Unpaired electrons are unbalanced electrical energy and these molecules "want" to find another electron to pair with. In their search for balanced energy, many of these free radicals steal an electron from already-paired matches, thus creating another free radical and propagating the problem. When these free radicals steal electrons from molecules found in our cell membranes, they often break apart paired molecules and disrupt metabolic processes. This process creates metabolic waste compounds called lipofuscins, which remain deposited in the cell and cause a darkening of the skin that we then call "age spots." When lipofuscin spots appear on the back of the hands, they are called "liver spots," and it is now believed that they are also deposited in the brain leading to neurological deterioration.

Free radicals are not unlike the promiscuous and conniving "bombshell" character that is found in many movie plots. In this classic Hollywood story, the ruthless and desperate single woman is always looking to "steal" a happily paired man from what is seemingly a blissful marriage to another woman. Maybe you've seen a movie or two like this, or maybe you've known some people like this in your life. Just as the forceful breakup of a marriage can cause havoc in a family, the damage caused by free radicals can create mayhem in your body.

Experts have reported that free radicals bombard every one of the 75 trillion cells of your body more than 10,000 times per day. Free radicals cause oxidation in our bodies. Oxidation is a word that describes the loss of electrons (remember that the free radicals are stealing them). Don't worry, we're not going to go into a big chemistry lesson. Instead, let's take a look at a classic example of an oxidation reaction, rust. When metal, especially iron, is left out in the elements, it rusts. The moisture in the air acts as a free radical and accelerates the process. Metal that has rusted becomes crumbly and falls apart, no longer moves the way it used to, and darkens in color. Sound familiar? This is similar to the process that occurs in our cells where the free radicals that we are exposed to cause "rusting" in our transport proteins that help move nutrients in and out of our cells, in our hormone receptors, and in the proteins that transcribe our genetic code.

Combine the information on incidence of free-radical exposure with the fact that it was reported that only 11 percent of Americans consume the recommended five-to-seven servings of antioxidant-rich fruits and vegetables, and no wonder we are noticing such a decline in our overall health! The fact that 89 percent of us fail to eat our vegetables is disgraceful. We really should know better. Most all of us can remember our mothers requiring us to finish whatever the green stuff on our plate was at dinner. Fruits and vegetables (especially the colorful ones) are rich in antioxidants. Antioxidants work to stabilize the free radicals and stop them from stealing electrons and causing damage. So by not eating your veggies and fruits, your body doesn't have enough antioxidants to absorb the free radicals. You have likely heard of antioxidants as they get a lot of press these days, and "green drinks" and antioxidant supplements have become very popular to augment one's diet. **Bottomline: Free radicals put your body at grave risk for cell destruction, degenerative diseases, endocrine disruption, premature aging, and mutation at the cellular level.**

Antioxidants quench and neutralize free radicals which, when left unchecked, will accelerate premature aging and overall destruction of your health. Even if you lived in the most pristine environment, the fact is that free radicals are formed naturally in our bodies by normal metabolic processes and are even used by our immune systems to fight pathogenic organisms. Every time you take a breath you are increasing your free-radical burden (but don't stop breathing)! Once again, we recommend that you balance adequate antioxidants and avoid situations that create excessive free radicals such as when the body is exposed to stress, pollution, chemicals, cigarette smoke, radiation, alcohol, high-fat foods, ozone, food additives, and fuel emissions.

NEUROENDOCRINE THEORY OF AGING

The Neuroendocrine Theory of Aging was developed in 1954 by Russian professor Vladimir Dilman and further revised by Ward Dean, MD. This theory states that aging is caused by a loss of sensitivity of the receptors in the hypothalamus as well as in the peripheral tissues to bind to neurotransmitters and hormones. Without these receptors working properly, the actions of neurotransmitters and hormones are altered significantly. In fact, the absence of a receptor renders the transmitter molecule completely ineffective. Do you have a junk drawer somewhere in your house that's full of keys that you no longer have the doors or locks for? Once upon a time, these keys were of vital importance

There are two types of diabetes and we often call them type 1 and type 2, (although we used to call them childhood onset and adult onset). In type 1 diabetes, the pancreas doesn't produce insulin. (Insulin is the hormone that allows the glucose to enter the cell to be used for energy.) The glucose stays in the blood and the cells starve. In type 2 diabetes, the pancreas produces enough insulin, but the cells don't recognize it anymore so the cells suffer from a similar state: they are starving for the glucose. In type 1 diabetics, you would see elevated blood glucose levels, but decreased blood insulin levels. In type 2 diabetics, their labs would reflect high levels of both blood glucose and insulin.

and allowed you access to whatever house or office or bike lock that you needed to get into, and you would have likely gone into a panic attack if you lost them or they were taken. Now the keys lie scattered across the bottom of a dirty drawer, useless and waiting for you to throw them out. The key is only as good as the lock it belongs to, and likewise a hormone is only as good as the receptor it binds to.

With age, our hormone and neurotransmitter receptors become altered and sometimes disappear altogether. You may already be familiar with this concept of resistance, as it's the primary mechanism that is responsible for type 2 diabetes. Insulin is a hormone and its primary function is to allow the cells of the body to use glucose for fuel. Every cell in the body has insulin receptors, and when insulin binds to those receptors, it allows our cells to take in glucose to use for energy. With insulin resistance, it's like the locks have been changed and the insulin can no longer fit into the receptor to activate it. Another place we see receptor resistance is in the case of the neurotransmitter serotonin. There is evidence that the serotonin receptors will reduce their activity, especially when flooded with serotonin,[5] as in the case of prolonged psychological stress and the use of selective serotonin reuptake inhibitors (SSRIs), a major class of antidepressant drugs that includes the seemingly ubiquitous Prozac. SSRIs prevent the serotonin from being broken down, which provides the synapse (area between the neurons) with an artificially high concentration of serotonin. This can dramatically affect the way we feel since serotonin is one of the major neurotransmitters that controls mood as well as sleep, sexuality, and appetite. Also, there is a relationship between type 2 diabetes and depression that has been well documented. It's possible that these conditions are seen in conjunction with one another because they are both caused by general receptor resistance.

What occurs with serotonin receptors in the brain and the gut, and insulin receptors in various tissues occurs with cortisol receptors, testosterone receptors, and other hormone receptors throughout the body. It is our estimate that in the not-too-distant future there will be an increased appreciation in the general medical community that cellular resistance and habituation is much more prevalent than previously believed. Just as we all know that "insulin resistance" is part of type 2 diabetes and the rising numbers of people suffering from this condition are largely responsible for the premature aging and disease in America, we will soon be discussing cortisol resistance due to chronic stress and adrenaline desensitization. As receptors become less responsive, it takes more and more of the activating substance to elicit a reaction. This is what causes the rise in insulin levels with diabetics and the drive to push further and further to get the same high for "adrenaline junkies." They are simply pushing to get more adrenaline because their receptors are desensitized. To get the same rush that you may have gotten from waterskiing a few years ago now requires skydiving or bungee jumping.

It's not just peripheral tissues that become less sensitive to hormone levels. Dilman and Dean described a process where the hypothalamus becomes desensitized or resistant to stimulation by testosterone, which results in the hypothalamus advising the pituitary to release more LH (leutinizing hormone). You should remember that the LH acts on the Leydig cells in the testicle to produce testosterone. This would likely result in an increase in testosterone production except that over time the Leydig cells become resistant to the LH and they ultimately produce less testosterone. It's all about these receptor molecules that are large and complicated proteins found on the cell membrane and how they fail to function properly as we age. These proteins may not be functioning properly due to glycation, cross-linking, free-radical damage, or just the fact that they are tired from all of the wear and tear they have endured.

The aging process is occurring regardless of how you look at it, or whose theory you subscribe to. In fact, most of these theories include aspects of each of the others, and they don't present themselves as mutually exclusive. Just as in any situation where there are multiple perspectives, the truth is usually somewhere in the middle and includes aspects from all observers. It is often said that the body has an innate wisdom, and the intricate systems and multiple levels of regulation leading to optimal testosterone levels are a perfect example of that wisdom; but along with that comes greater opportunity for a disruption in the process resulting in decreased androgen levels. Between problems with the hypothalamus or in the pituitary, damage to the testes or resistance in the peripheral tissues, it seems like there are so many things that can go wrong! Just like with toys or electronics, the more moving parts and the more complex the system, the greater the opportunity for there to be a problem.

Are you getting depressed thinking about all of the aging that is going on in your body as you are reading this? Are you afraid you might wake up tomorrow and admit to your wife, "Honey, my hormone receptors are acting up again"? Or maybe, "I just can't handle this constant barrage of free radicals!"? Well then, don't just sit there on the couch and passively let it all happen. Sure, there's some truth to the old adage that ignorance is bliss, and in fact you may have been happier when you could eat a basket of french fries and drink a pitcher of beer with your buddies and not think about or even know the damage that you were causing to your body. As you educate yourself, you'll find that you may pay more attention to labels in the grocery store, and start to ask more questions about where things come from and what is in them. This awareness will pay off if you stick to your guns and make the changes you need to make. You'll feel better, look better, and . . . perform better. So, let's get started. It's finally time to take action!

NOTES

1. Klatz, R. and R. Goldman, *The Official Anti-Aging Revolution: Stop the Clock, Time is On Your Side* (Basic Health Publications, 2007).

2. Rudman, D., A.G. Feller, H.S. Nograj, "Effects of human growth hormone in men over 60 years old," *New England Journal of Medicine* (1990) 323:1–6.

3. Johnson, R.K. and C. Frary, "Choose beverages and foods to moderate your intake of sugars: the 2000 dietary guidelines for Americans–what's all the fuss about?" *J Nutr* (2001) Oct, 131(10):2766S–2771S.

    4. McPherson, J.D., B.H. Shilton, D.J. Walton, "Role of fructose in glycation and cross-linking of proteins," *Biochemistry* (1988) 27:1901–7.

    5. Smolin, B., E. Klein, Y. Levy, D. BenShachar, "Major depression as a disorder of serotonin resistance: inference from diabetes mellitus type II," *Int J Neuropsychopharmacol* (2007) Dec; 10(6):839–50; E-pub 2007 Jan 25.

CHAPTER 7

Testing and Monitoring Hormone Levels

Diagnostics are important in any field whether it is mechanics, engineering, construction, or health care, and they are especially important when it comes to your health. You wouldn't take your car into the mechanic and tell him, "It's making a dinging sound, let's replace the head gasket and see if that helps." Likewise, you shouldn't try new medications or medical procedures without investigating what is causing the problem in the first place. The importance of proper assessment of a situation before deciding what action should be taken is possibly summed up best in the common saying in carpentry: "measure twice, cut once." Okay, with health care costs the way they are today, you probably can't afford to measure twice, and we wouldn't ask you to, but taking the time and resources to measure your hormone levels and to take a look at other important tests is invaluable to your health.

Conventional reasons for laboratory assessment are to allow you and your doctor to see changes in your health **before** symptoms occur, give you **additional information** about what may be causing the symptoms you are having, to help formulate your **treatment** plan, or help to evaluate or **track your response** to a treatment. There's another reason to test your body chemistry, and that's just to have a baseline to compare future lab values to. Even if you feel 100 percent healthy as you are reading this, we recommend you get tested so you will have a point of reference if things change. Lab values are relative, and knowing how things have changed over time is invaluable information. We believe that good preventative or proactive medicine starts way before you get "sick," which means both before you have symptoms and before you have signs. Proactive medicine is the alternative to the reactive medicine that is largely practiced in this country. The point is, don't wait until you find yourself in the ER, or taking a bunch of pharmaceuticals if you don't have to. Most (or at least many) of you probably go to the dentist to have your teeth cleaned to **prevent** cavities. We're suggesting you treat your whole body as well as you treat your teeth. Get yourself checked before there is a problem. The big question is not whether or not you should test, but rather what to test and how to do it.

So far we have talked primarily about testosterone, and testosterone is of utmost importance when it comes to men's health. Testing testosterone levels is a primary concern with andropause, especially when we are considering bio-identical hormone replacement therapy. Free-testosterone levels are the most useful since it shows us what is actually available to the tissues. There are also several other hormones that play a role in your well-being; it's hard to isolate just one hormone without discussing its interactions with the others. Progesterone and estrogen are important to test because of their roles in prostate health and especially because of the relationship between estrogen and testosterone. DHEA is a stress hormone produced by the adrenal glands, but is also a precursor molecule that can turn into estrogen or testosterone, so it's important to monitor. And cortisol, the primary stress hormone that is produced in your adrenal glands, is a big part of your fight-or-flight response and sometimes plays a role in suppression of testosterone.

By now, you may have read about many symptoms associated with hormone imbalance and realized that it's entirely likely that many of the problems you've been noticing creeping into your life may be attributed to a less-than-optimal testosterone level or imbalance in your estrogen/progesterone ratio. Call it aging, andropause, or just an inability to rise to the occasion as often as you used to. You are not feeling like your "young self." Maybe you are still performing well, but are on the threshold of a newer, healthier lifestyle and want to know exactly how much you've been affected by the less-than-perfect diet and infrequent exercise program that you are now leaving in the past. We recommend that you start this process by finding a physician who works with bio-identical hormones and can guide you in not only testing your hormones, but also monitoring other parameters to ensure that you are being safe and effective with your treatment. You may already have a medical doctor, naturopathic doctor,

Resources for finding a hormone-savvy practitioner near you:

- American College for Advancement in Medicine (ACAM)—www.acam.org

- American Association of Naturopathic Physicians (AANP)—www.naturopathic.org

- John R. Lee, MD—www.drjohnlee.com

- The International Academy of Compounding Pharmacists (IACP)—www.iacprx.org

- The Institute for Functional Medicine (IFM)—www.functionalmedicine.org

- American Academy of Anti-Aging Medicine (A4M)—www.worldhealth.net

physician's assistant, a chiropractor, nurse practitioner, or pharmacist who is well-versed in the intricate world of hormones. If not, we have listed a couple of resources where you can look for a qualified professional who can assist you with thorough testing as well as guide you with a treatment plan that may include bio-identical hormone replacement therapy. Of course, the point of this book is to help you be as informed as possible when you are working with your physician or any healthcare provider because you are the most important player in the management of your health. Your physicians or team of providers are just there to assist you. It is important for all of us to remember that a healthcare provider is supposed to provide health care, not just sick care. True health care should include wellness care. Furthermore, it's important to remember that your physicians are hired professionals working for you, and just as you wouldn't tolerate an electrician, plumber, or mechanic who doesn't listen to your needs, you should find a doctor to work with who will give you the care you want.

Our bodies are very dynamic and many things are changing all the time. Sometimes that works to our advantage. We may be so sick one day that we can't get out of bed and by the very next afternoon can hardly recall that we weren't feeling well. Even when we are well, our systems are constantly changing and adjusting, establishing and reestablishing equilibrium. Hormone levels fluctuate throughout the day, week, and month so measured levels can vary significantly depending on when you submit your sample. We like to explain to our patients that lab tests are like snapshots or pictures of what is going on in the body at that exact moment. Just as you can take a picture of an airplane as it flies by, you know that the plane was only in that exact place for that brief moment or it would have fallen out of the sky! Some testing methods are better for monitoring the changing lab values than others, just as some testing methods give you a better overall average. There are many reasons why you and your physician may choose one testing method over another.

SERUM

Serum is the fluid that can be separated from the red and white blood cells in blood. Though serum looks clear (not cloudy) and yellowish in color, somewhat resembling urine, it has many proteins, hormones, and nutrients in it. After blood is drawn from your vein, it is spun in a machine called a centrifuge and the blood cells separate from the serum because they have more mass than the serum. Hormones can be found in the serum, but the problem is that most of them are bound to carrier proteins like SHBG, CBG, and albumin (another carrier protein that is less specific and binds less strongly). Hormones are lipid soluble, which means that they dissolve in fats, and serum is an aqueous or water-like environment. Like oil and water, they don't mix well. Many tests look for the total amount of the hormone in the body, regardless of whether or not that hormone is bound to a protein (rendering it unavailable to tissues). These total hormone levels are commonly run by conventional physicians. Though the total hormone levels matter, the most important thing is what your tissues can actually

Total testosterone level is like looking at a bank statement that combines your investments, savings, and checking accounts and the money in your pocket all into one number. It may look like you have plenty of money, but chances are the majority of that money isn't available for you to use very readily. The hormone bound to the SHBG is like money in a mutual fund; you count it as an asset, it belongs to you, but it's not very easy to access it. There is a weaker bond between the hormones and albumin, so these hormones are more like your savings account. This is money you have put away, but you can transfer it to your checking account with minimal effort. Only about two to three percent of all testosterone in the body is "free" or unbound to carrier proteins. This is like the money in your pocket; you can spend it easily to grab a cup of coffee.

access to use. It doesn't matter if you have several million dollars in investments, if you don't have five dollars in your pocket or your checking account, you can't even buy lunch!

When the hormone is bound to a carrier protein, it is not available to bind to receptors in target tissues, and so, in essence, is just a reservoir of hormone that can't be used. Testosterone is tested in serum using several different methods. Some of the methods are used for screening purposes only because they aren't sensitive enough to diagnose patients with hypogonadism. These less expensive tests are often used initially to see if you are in the ballpark before going on to more sensitive and less economical testing. In almost all cases, the free testosterone level is calculated from the total testosterone level and the SHBG level using an equation, although it is sometimes determined by a process called equilibrium dialysis, where they use a process to separate bound hormones from free hormones and give you the percentage of the total hormone that is available to bind to receptors (free). SHBG levels are tested in serum and are needed to calculate the free testosterone level. There is a test that can measure free testosterone levels directly; however, it is much more expensive, many labs don't offer it, and there is some controversy with how well it correlates to the calculated free testosterone especially in men with low SHBG concentrations.[1] The Free Androgen Index (FAI) is a calculation done with measured total testosterone levels and SHBG levels and is a rough estimate of the free testosterone that is available to the tissues. A healthy FAI level should be 0.8–1.2. Generally, men with an FAI of 0.7 or lower are considered hypogonadal. As stated earlier, it's difficult to look at just one hormone and see the whole picture as they all play a role. There is no serum test for "free progesterone," yet we know that progesterone is important in protecting the prostate and, therefore, is useful to look at. Like the other steroid hormones, progesterone likes fat, not water, and is bound to carrier proteins in the blood. You can test for progesterone in serum, but you don't really know how much of that is available to tissues. There are several forms of estrogen found in our bodies, and estradiol or E2 is the primary circulating form. Actually, E2 stays in approximate equilibrium with estrone (E1) and the third form, estriol (E3), is the most minor of players. Estradiol is the form of estrogen that we recommend you measure when it comes to testing. Estradiol has a lot in common with testosterone. It binds to the same binding proteins (SHBG and albumin), and the same measurement processes and similar calculations are used to determine the free and total amounts; however, estrogen is rarely discussed in terms of "free" and "total" values the way that testosterone is.

There are some significant downfalls to serum testing. Many of the hormones have a diurnal rhythm (or a pattern) throughout the day. Testosterone and cortisol are both highest in the morning, so if you are testing via serum, you are best with a morning blood draw so the "picture" you are taking is when the levels are at their best. Specifically, cortisol levels reach their peak approximately thirty minutes after you wake up. Of course, this isn't always very convenient for people since to have serum testing you have to be in a lab or doctor's office to have your blood drawn. In very few cases can you get up and make it to a blood draw station within the first hour after you wake up. Some people have difficult veins and find that every time they need a blood test, the phlebotomist sets off to find their vein like the proverbial needle in a haystack, not to mention the fact that many people are just plain scared of needles. Even big, strong men often get queasy or lightheaded when they are exposed to a needle or their own blood. In fact, the first patient I (S. Wood) ever had pass out on me during a blood draw was a six-feet-and-one-inch, athletic, 28-year-old who was an avid extreme sports enthusiast. Skydiving, snowboarding, and bungee jumping didn't alarm him, but that little needle in his arm sure unnerved him. When you are talking about testing cortisol (a stress hormone), then this type of reaction isn't just unpleasant for the patient, but will literally affect the values you are monitoring! Studies have shown that venipuncture alone causes enough of a stress response in many people to stimulate cortisol production, resulting in artificially elevated cortisol levels.[2]

We haven't gotten to the chapter on what you can do with all of this information, but it's important for you to know that if you are deficient, supplementing with bio-identical hormone replacement therapy (BHRT) may make a huge difference. There are several ways to go about supplementing hormones (and there will be more on that later), but one very common way of administering hormones is through a transdermal cream. The reason we mention this now is because although topical hormones have been shown to be very effective in managing patients' symptoms and certainly have a significant effect in the body, hormones that are administered through the skin don't affect serum levels very much. When the hormone is applied to the skin, the free hormones are absorbed directly into the fat layer beneath the skin (called the subcutaneous fat). Red blood cells (RBCs) passing through the areas' capillary beds bind loosely to the hormones. Remember that hormones are lipophilic, which means that they like to be near fatty compounds and not near watery compounds. Cell membranes are made of fatty acids and cholesterol, and so the hormone fits right in. There are a number of different ways that molecules can bind or associate with one another. You may remember this from chemistry class years ago, but some molecular bonds are like glue and require some significant effort to break apart, whereas other molecular relationships are more like holding hands so it is not difficult for them to disassociate. The connection between the hormone and the blood cell is not very secure, so the hormones are released from the RBCs easily in target tissues.[3] Remember that when a test is run on serum, the blood cells have been separated from the serum by the centrifuge, taking the hormones bound to their membranes with them. Even though the relationship between these hormones and the red blood cells they are hitching a ride on is weak, the process of extracting the hormones from the red blood cells isn't very easy to do, alters the results of the test, and is expensive. So when in the blood stream, hormones are either bound to their respective carrier proteins (like SHBG), to albumin, loosely to the RBCs, or unbound in the serum. Remember that your system is dynamic, and though it's easy to think of the hormone as neatly "filed" in one of these places for simplification purposes, the reality is that they are constantly moving between these various states. When we take hormones orally, they must be bound to proteins to be absorbed from the GI tract, so the lab values reflect an increase in total hormone level, but the value of the free hormone remains relatively unchanged.

Some of the drawbacks to using serum for testing testosterone and the other steroid hormones are the intricate calculation and increased expense, the fact that the values can't be used to accurately monitor some BHRT therapies (because it doesn't accurately measure available hormone levels), and you still have to get stuck with a needle! There must be some reasons to test for hormones in serum if it's still the most common way they are tested, right? If you are already drawing blood to run other tests and you want to get a rough idea of whether or not there is a problem, serum values can be useful. Most doctors use serum to monitor many of the body's functions, from liver enzymes to cholesterol levels, and so they are most accustomed to looking at serum to assess what is going on. Blood testing is typically the "gold standard" for everything having to do with body chemistry and so many doctors stick to serum testing simply due to convention.

URINE

There are many doctors who prefer to test for hormones in urine. This is usually done in a 24-hour urine collection. Because you collect your urine for an entire 24-hour period, the issue of circadian rhythm is more or less eliminated because you are looking at the average amount of the hormone produced in a 24-hour period. Urine tests are relatively economical because you can test for so many different primary and secondary hormones as well as their metabolites, which are the various breakdown products that come from the primary and secondary hormones (intermediates that are part of the synthesis process, but have relatively few primary responsibilities in the body). When a hormone is metabolized by the liver, it can be transformed into several different products that are then excreted in the urine. Before they are excreted, these products are present in the body for a period of time and can affect tissues. Some metabolites have been implicated in higher incidences of cancer. For example, there has been a lot of research done on the various metabolites of estrogen. One metabolite, 2-hydroxyestrone, has been shown to inhibit cancer growth, while another one, 16-a-hydroxyestrone, has been determined to encourage tumor development. There are many labs that measure these metabolites and then give a ratio of one to the other that can provide some information on risk of estrogen-sensitive cancers, although the there are conflicting opinions in the literature about whether or not these compounds are really affecting cancer. While the measurement of these metabolites of hormones is one of the "pros" for urine testing because of some of the unique information it provides, there are many factors that can alter the production of metabolites rendering it difficult to determine exactly how accurately they represent the amount of hormone that is available to the tissues. Our blood is "filtered" in our livers where hormones are modified to be more water soluble so that they can be excreted. The kidneys are then responsible for removing these water soluble compounds from our blood and eliminating them in the urine (which is mostly water). Impaired renal function (renal refers to your kidney) or dysfunction in your liver can alter the amount of a given metabolite that you produce, regardless of the amount of hormone you had in the first place. And similarly to serum testing, hormone levels in urine don't accurately reflect the bioavailable hormone levels when topical replacement therapy is employed.

Collecting your urine for 24 hours turns out to be challenging for many patients because it means that you have to collect every drop of your urine for a 24-hour period. It doesn't sound too difficult at first, but no one wants to be carting around a gallon jug full of urine at work, and even if you do the test on the weekend, you are still tied to the house all day because you certainly aren't going to want to be at the ballpark with your urine bottle, and never mind how easy it is to get up in the middle of the night, still half asleep and miss a sample. Still, many would prefer it to a needle, but these aren't the only two options.

SALIVA

Saliva is produced in (and secreted from) salivary glands located in your mouth. Blood is filtered through the acinar cells in the salivary glands, and during this process, the hormones that are bound to large protein complexes such as SHBG and albumin find that they are not able to pass through the cell membranes. The hormones that are loosely bound to the red blood cells pass relatively easily through the glands just as they are easily absorbed by tissues, and this results in only the free or unbound (bioavailable) hormones being able to make it into saliva. The saliva glands are like nature's sieve, automatically screening out the hormones that your tissues can't use. Remember that the hormones that are bound to the large proteins don't fit into the receptors, so they are inactive. As long as the hormones are bound to those proteins, they are essentially in storage, like money in a mutual fund or CD.

Salivary hormone levels are significantly lower than you would find in serum because only approximately one to two percent of hormones are nonprotein bound.[4] Essentially this difference between saliva- and serum-tested values is the difference between free and total hormone levels. For this reason, dosage of hormone replacement therapy must certainly be determined based on what kind of test was done to ensure that you aren't given too much hormone. This is an important point because many studies that have been done utilize serum testing since (as we've mentioned) serum is the conventional way to test and monitor most functions of the body. If a hormone study is done using serum testing, then the dosages used in the study may not be safe because the values from the test aren't likely to reflect the amount delivered to the tissues.

Testing hormone levels is typically done for two reasons. The first is to see what your baseline lab values are. This is usually done based on some symptoms that indicate to you or your doctor that you may have a hormone imbalance. The second reason to test for hormones is to monitor treatment that you are receiving to ensure that you are getting enough of what you need to create optimum health without an excess of anything. As we learned in chapter 4, there are as many problems with too much hormones just as there can be with too little.

Saliva testing is very easy for anyone to do, and enables the patient to take samples at various time throughout the day. Remember that many hormones have a daily rhythm, and by testing at various times you not only pinpoint what the problem is, but when it is occurring! Urine tests give you the total for an entire day, which is like a panoramic picture as opposed to a quick snapshot, but if you have cortisol levels that are extremely high in the evening, but then on the low end for the rest of the day, they may average out and be in range with a 24-hour test. With saliva, you usually provide four samples, one within thirty minutes of waking, one before lunch, one before dinner, and a final sample before bed. This gives you much more detail. Have you ever flipped back and forth between high-definition and regular TV during a football game? Big difference, right? Just as you want to have the clearest, most detailed view of your team on Sunday, you also want the best view of your hormone levels. An optimal cortisol profile, for example, is highest in the morning and then gradually declines throughout the day. If you looked at two patients, one with a relatively healthy cortisol profile and one who had an extreme spike in the evening, they could have similar numbers with a 24-hour urine test. If a serum test was done around 1:00 P.M., they would have nearly identical "snapshots."

The two patients profiled in figure 7.1 have exactly the same daily average and daily total, yet Patient A has an extremely out-of-range evening cortisol value, while Patient B has adequate cortisol levels and the curve fits the optimal pattern. In addition to giving you a more detailed picture, providing a saliva sample takes only a few minutes, doesn't involve anything sharp or a large jug of urine, and gives you the most accurate assessment of your treatment, especially if you are using topical hormones. Cortisol was the first hormone to be studied in saliva and is still one of the only saliva tests that many conventional doctors perform. For example, Quest Diagnostics, a large national lab, provides a saliva cortisol test, but not a saliva test, for any of the sex hormones. These hormones are very similar in structure, and can all be found in their bioavailable form in saliva.

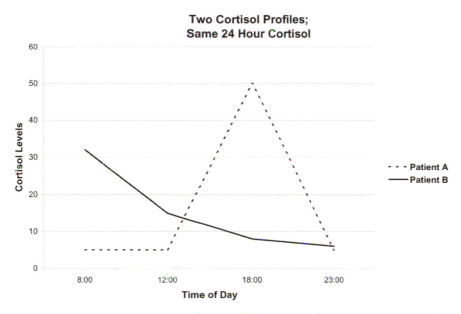

Figure 7.1 These two patients have the same daily average of cortisol output, yet wildly different scenerios going on in their bodies.

Though we've tried to present the multiple options in hormone testing, we prefer saliva testing for the reasons we've listed above: it's easy, it's economical, and it's accurate. In our opinion, saliva wins in all three categories. We recommend that you get your estradiol, progesterone, testosterone, DHEA, and cortisol levels checked. Proper cortisol assessment really requires that you look at several measurements throughout the day, as their rhythms tell you as much information about adrenal function as the values alone do. Morning, noon, evening, and night values are preferable. You probably have a pretty good idea from the first several chapters about why we recommend you test testosterone levels, and we've explained the importance of estrogen and its balance with progesterone when it comes to prostate health. We covered the role of cortisol, but we've not explained the role that DHEA plays in all of this.

DHEA is a hormone that is produced by the adrenal glands, although it comes from the zona reticularis, which is a different compartment of the adrenal gland than where cortisol is produced. DHEA is an androgen hormone and is a prohormone, or a precursor to estrogen and testosterone. It is secreted during a stress response along with cortisol, and it is believed to calm emotions, increase alertness, help deal with stress, and improve memory. Much like testosterone, DHEA declines with age, beginning at approximately age 25–30. DHEA exists in the body in two forms, the free as well as the sulphated form, which is referred to as DHEA-S. Because it must be desulfated to be biologically active, it is the DHEA, not the DHEA-S, that should be measured to get an idea of accurate available levels in the body. Like the other hormones we've discussed, DHEA can most accurately be measured in saliva.

	Pros	Cons
Serum	• Conventional doctors are used to this method • Can be done at same time as other blood work	• Requires a needle and a trip to the lab • Provides info for one point in time • Doesn't change with transdermal supplementation, can't monitor topical treatment • Values reflect total, not free levels of the hormones • Can be expensive
Urine	• Looks at all metabolites, provides info on pathways • Gives overall picture for whole day, not snapshot • Can be done at home, very little stress • Economical	• Affected by liver and kidney function • Requires 24 hours of urine collection in a large jug
Saliva	• Easy to do at home, no stress • Provides multiple data points to follow diurnal rhythms • Can be used to monitor topical treatment • Provides only bioavailable (free) hormone levels • Is inexpensive	• Possible difficulty with certain diseases such as Sjogrens (an autoimmune disease in moisture producing glands) • Restricted to steroid hormones, and not protein hormones such as insulin or thyroid hormones • Saliva can be contaminated by presence of topical hormones on lips or hands.

Figure 7.2 Pros and Cons of testing.

ADDITIONAL LAB VALUES YOU SHOULD BE WATCHING

One of the reasons we recommend you do your hormone testing through a doctor or other healthcare provider who is familiar with hormones is so that you have the option to treat any deficiencies with bio-identical hormones, but also because there are a number of conditions that accompany testosterone deficiency that should be looked at in addition to hormone levels. In the event that you do begin a supplementation plan, there are also a few tests that you will want to monitor.

We have already talked about SHBG because its measurement is important if you are measuring testosterone in serum. You must have the SHBG level to determine the free androgen index because total testosterone levels alone don't give you much useful information. If you are testing for hormones in either urine or saliva, then knowing the SHBG level may not be necessary. SHBG can function as an estrogen amplifier because its production is increased in the presence of estrogen, but it binds to testosterone more tightly than to estrogen, which potentially displaces estrogen that was bound to the protein, leaving more binding sites for testosterone and further pushing free testosterone levels lower. As a result, you end up with even more estrogen than you started with, and less testosterone.

Your prostate specific antigen (PSA) should be tested before the initiation of treatment with hormones (and monitored throughout). Like testosterone, there are several different ways to measure PSA. The total PSA is a more sensitive test, meaning that if you were having a prostate problem, then the PSA would be elevated. There are few false negatives. Total PSA is measured in ng/mL, whereas the free PSA is a **percentage** of the PSA that isn't bound to proteins in the blood. The free PSA is more specific, meaning that fewer patients without cancer test positive (fewer false positives). A free PSA of less than 25 percent is more specific to prostate cancer. You can start out running a total and then have your doctor add a free level if the total level is ele-

Sensitivity and specificity are two parameters that we often use when referring to testing methods. What's the difference? Well, sensitivity refers to how likely the test is to detect whatever condition you are looking for. With a sensitive test, you could use a **negative result to rule out** a disease. Specificity refers to how likely a positive result is to correlate with the disease or condition you are testing for. So, with a specific test, you can **diagnose a disease with a positive** result. Imagine you are trying to record a lecture or speech with an audio recorder. You want to pick up all the sounds from the speech clearly without too much background noise. If your microphone is sensitive, then you are likely to hear everything that is said but have some additional background noises that aren't coming from the speaker, such as sounds from the audience. If your microphone is specific, then it will pick up only sounds from the presenter and rule out additional sounds, but you may not be able to clearly hear everything that is said.

vated. Of course, monitoring your prostate in general is a good idea since prostate cancer is the most common cancer in men in the United States, and is responsible for the second-highest number of cancer deaths (only lung cancer kills more people).

Just a brief recap for those of you who haven't had an anatomy class in a while (or maybe not at all). The prostate is a small gland located just below the bladder. The urethra passes through it on its way to the penis. The prostate secretes fluid that, along with the sperm from the testicles and seminal fluid from the seminal vesicles, makes up semen. It also plays a role in preventing urine from entering the urethra during an ejaculation, like a cop directing traffic at a busy intersection. An elevated PSA is certainly not diagnostic for prostate cancer; not only is it produced by some other tissues (though in much, much smaller amounts), it is also not produced exclusively by cancer. PSA is part of the seminal fluid that the prostate produces and is believed to play a role in helping the sperm swim freely and assisting them in breaking through cervical mucus to gain entry into the uterus, which enhances fertility.

An elevated PSA level simply indicates that the prostate cells are active, so increased PSA levels can indicate recent ejaculation, a recent digital rectal exam, prostate infection or inflammation, or the very common benign prostatic hyperplasia (BPH). PSA is a blood test, though it often is accompanied by a digital rectal exam (DRE) where a physician uses his or her finger to feel the prostate for increased size, irregularity, or nodularity. As you have probably guessed by the name, the best way to reach the prostate is through the rectum and this procedure could possibly be single-handedly responsible for why so many men refuse to go to a doctor! While a PSA and DRE are often used in tandem to diagnose prostate problems, the PSA is a simple blood test and we would encourage you to make sure that you are having this test done on a regular basis regardless of whether or not you are supplementing hormones. If you are going to take testosterone however, it is necessary that you have your PSA checked **prior** to starting treatment. While we explained in previous chapters that testosterone doesn't cause prostate cancer, it may exacerbate it if the condition already exists. Remember that it is important to consult with your doctor prior to starting any new therapy. You should always keep your primary care provider informed of all supplements, therapies and treatments that you are considering so that they can provide you with optimal care and possibly alert you to any side effects or interactions with any existing condition you may have.

Tests for Optimal Health

Saliva:

- Free testosterone
- Estradiol
- Progesterone
- DHEA
- Cortisol (4 times/day)

Blood:

- Free and total PSA
- Fasting insulin
- Fasting glucose
- Hemoglobin A1c
- Fractionated lipid panel
- Cardio C-reactive protein
- Homocysteine
- Fibrinogen
- 25-hydroxycholecalciferol (Vitamin D)
- Food allergy test

Urine:

- 24-hour iodine challenge

Polysomnography:

- Sleep apnea screening

Because metabolic syndrome is so closely tied to testosterone in men, you may want to look at your fasting glucose and fasting insulin levels to see how your body is metabolizing glucose or sugar. Metabolic syndrome is a pre-diabetic condition that includes insulin resistance as well as elevated triglycerides, elevated cholesterol, increased visceral abdominal fat, and raised blood pressure, all severely increasing your risk of heart disease. Cholesterol and triglycerides are both part of a basic lipid panel that can be run by any lab, or you and your doctor may want to run a more specific test that includes lipoprotein(a) and other fractionated lipids like the VAP (vertical auto profile). Tests such as the VAP are much more specific than just telling you cholesterol and triglyceride levels, and may increase the ability to predict heart disease from 40 percent to 90 percent! Additional risk factors for heart disease are C-reactive protein (CRP), fibrinogen, and homocysteine levels. Most of these tests (insulin, glucose, lipids, CRP) should be tested in your serum, and you will need to be fasting for 9 to12 hours before the blood is drawn. In most cases, you will simply make an appointment to have your blood drawn in the morning before breakfast, and keep yourself from raiding the refrigerator at midnight. These labs should accompany your initial hormone test to help you and your doctor look at the big picture, and so you can both know just how far-reaching the effects of decreased testosterone levels are.

Hemoglobin A1c is another blood test that can give you a broader picture of what is happening with your blood sugar. Have you ever let your child try to eat a candied apple? Or maybe you've had this experience yourself. It's almost impossible not to get that caramel all over your face, hands, and lap because sugar sticks to everything. The same thing happens in your blood. When your blood glucose levels are elevated, the sugar sticks to blood vessels, blood cells, etc. We call this process glycosylation or glycation, and you may remember this from the cross-linking theory of aging. One of the many things that the glucose will stick to is hemoglobin, a protein that carries oxygen in your red blood cells. If you test for the glycosylated hemoglobin, it will give an approximation of how high blood sugars have been over the 120-day life pan of the red blood cell, so this is one blood test that doesn't just give you a "snapshot," but tells you a longer story.

It's not just testosterone and DHEA that fall with age. Growth hormone levels decline significantly as well over the years. By the age of 60, it's estimated that at least 30 percent of apparently healthy men have lower-than-optimal levels. Sound familiar? So, how do you know if your growth hormone levels are low? HGH (human growth hormone) levels vary dramatically throughout the day, and the hormone remains active in the bloodstream for only a few minutes after it's been released, so it's not a very easy hormone to test for directly. When the liver takes in HGH, it is converted into several other substances, one of which is called insulin-like growth factor 1 (IGF-1). As you may guess from its name, IGF-1 has a structure very similar to insulin, but for our purposes it is most useful as a stable biomarker of approximate growth hormone levels. Because the levels of IGF-1 do not fluctuate significantly throughout the day, it is used as a screening test and a way to monitor growth hormone therapy. If you are interested in knowing if your growth hormone levels are declining, this is a simple blood test that can be run with your other tests. Knowing what your IGF-1 levels are is useful even if you don't plan on taking growth hormone supplements as there are many natural ways to stimulate HGH production.

Vitamin D is a fat-soluble vitamin that we get from cold-water fish and is often fortified in (added to) milk and dairy products, but our primary source of vitamin D is from the sun. Our body can synthesize the bioactive form of vitamin D with the help of UVB rays found in sunshine. Unfortunately, there are a couple of factors that keep this from happening as often we need it. The first is the angle of the sun. The sun must be at an angle greater than 45 degrees for the UVB rays to reach us. For many of us in the upper latitudes of the country, this only occurs for a few months of the year. Even during the summer months when the sun is at an adequately high place in the sky, many of us don't spend much time outside, and when we do we are often wearing sunscreen. People with increased melanin or darker complexions require longer sun exposures to produce the same amounts of the vitamin. You are probably thinking, "What is this? Doctors advocating sun exposure? But I thought I was supposed to stay out of the sun to prevent skin cancer!" Well, of course you should be cautious about skin cancers. Melanomas are extremely dangerous, but there needs to be a balance where we can manufacture enough vitamin D and not overexpose ourselves. There's that word **balance** again.

There are a couple of different forms of vitamin D in our systems. The sunlight transforms a precursor into cholecalciferol, which is also referred to as vitamin D3. (Another form of vitamin D is found in plant sources, and is called ergocalciferol or vitamin D2). The vitamin D3 that is created in the skin is hydroxylated (just a fancy word to mean that an enzyme adds an oxygen molecule to it) in the liver to form 25-hydroxycholcalciferol (we'll refer to it as 25(OH)D3 for short). Though this form is hydroxylated again in the kidney to create another form (called 1,25-dihydrocholecalciferol), and it is this form that is biologically active. The most prevalent form of the vitamin, and therefore the most accurate to measure to determine levels of the vitamin in the body, is the 25(OH)D3 form. Although vitamin D is created from cholesterol like other steroid hormones, and looks and acts very much like a steroid hormone, there isn't yet a test developed to look at vitamin D levels in saliva, and therefore, serum levels of 25(OH)D3 are the most effective tests. Keep in mind that when we say "steroid" here, we are simply referring to the fact that it has a ring structure and comes from cholesterol. If you haven't studied much chemistry, this may not make much sense to you, but because the word steroid is casually used to refer to substances that bodybuilders and athletes use, we don't want you to mistakenly think vitamin D will "pump you up."

So, why test vitamin D levels? Vitamin D binds to receptors found in tissues throughout the body and has effects that are very far-reaching and can be cancer protective, enhance immunity, prevent osteoporosis, control hypertension, and protect against type 2 diabetes through its ability to impair insulin synthesis and secretion.[5] Unlike the PSA, which we strongly recommend you have done prior to any hormone replacement, vitamin D levels are not imperative to treatment. They are simply an additional factor in your health that you can monitor and maintain. The relationship between vitamin D and androgen hormones such as testosterone is not direct, but they do have something in common as a deficiency in either is likely to cause or promote metabolic syndrome in men.

In addition to sex hormones and cortisol, which we highly recommend you have tested, screening your thyroid hormone is a good idea as well. The thyroid gland is located just below the Adam's apple in men and is responsible for pro-ducing a hormone that helps control the way cells metabolize proteins, fats, and carbohydrates. It also helps you generate heat. Just like many of the other hormones, thyroid hormone is bound to a transport protein called thyroxin binding globulin (TBG) when in the blood. The primary screening test for thyroid disease isn't to test for thyroid hormone at all, but to test for thyroid stimulating hormone (TSH), which is a hormone that is produced by the pituitary that in turn, as its name suggests, stimulates the thyroid to produce thyroid hormone. The thyroid produces a hormone called thyroxine (T4), which is named for the fact that it uses 4 molecules of iodine. In your peripheral tissues, the T4 is converted into triiodothyronine (T3) by removing one of the iodine molecules (hence the name T3). T3 is actually the more bioactive form, although there is significantly more T4 found in circulation. We recommend you monitor your TSH, as well as the unbound forms of both thyroid hormones—free T3 and free T4—for optimal initial assessment of thyroid function. If these tests indicate that there is a problem, you and your physician may want to take a look and see if you have any thyroid antibodies, which are your body's own immune cells that may be attacking your thyroid erroneously. Though we see thyroid disease more commonly in women, there are many men who are suffering from this problem and are often overlooked.

What do you know about iodine? Your mother may have used it as an antiseptic to clean scrapes and cuts when you were a kid, or you may vaguely remember it associated with salt for some reason. A survey of 3,000 Americans found that 95 percent of them were iodine deficient.[6] Iodine is used in all parts of your body including breast tissue, salivary glands, sweat glands, stomach lining, ovarian tissue, testicular tissue, heart, and liver, but is most important to thyroid function. In the 1920s, iodine was added to salt to provide us with the minimal dose that would prevent goiter (enlarged thyroid) and cretinism (a problem with proper brain development in babies) because our soil had been depleted of iodine and we were therefore not getting enough of it in our food. Iodinized salt and iodine used in breads as a rising agent provided (for the most part) the very minimal recommended daily allowance (RDA) of 150 micrograms that we need to prevent overt thyroid disease. As time went on, though, we stopped using as much salt due to its adverse effects on heart conditions; many people switched to sea salt that was non-iodinized, and we started using bromine instead of iodine in our breads. Bromine (which we find in other sources such as soda and cigarettes) is an element that is found in the same column on the periodic table and competes with iodine in the body. The use of bromine and other elements from that column, including chlorine and fluoride, have exacerbated the iodine deficiency. Analysis of the Japanese diet has indicated that they ingest an average of 13.8 mg of iodine (note that that is milligrams, we were previously talking micrograms). For those of you who aren't science people, that means that the Japanese are getting 13.8 mg to our approximate 0.15 mg. Sure enough, studies find that they have a much lower incidence of breast cancer and thyroid disease.[7]

As you can see, iodine plays a very important role in your health, and not only in your thyroid. And it's easy to test your levels to see if you, like so many Americans, are deficient. The best way to test iodine levels is with a urine spot test and 24-hour urine challenge. This means a first-morning urine sample is taken, after which 50 mg of iodine is ingested and then urine is collected for 24 hours. A small amount of the 24-hour total is then poured into a small sample bottle and the two samples are sent to the lab. The level of deficiency is based on the percentage of the 50 mg of iodine that you "spill" into your urine. If your tissues are deficient, they will hold onto the iodine and less of it will be excreted in your urine. Like the urine test for hormones, or any 24-hour urine collection, this test involves a big jug of urine that you fill. This is certainly a drawback to this test, just as it is with any 24-hour hormone test, but urine collection is really the "gold standard" with iodine testing.

This book is about hormones and that's certainly a large enough subject for a couple of books, but we would like to suggest a couple of additional obstacles that may exist between you and optimal health. While we are talking about testing, we want to bring to your attention a couple of tests that you may not know are out there. The first is a food allergy test. When you think of food allergies, you probably remember some kid in elementary school who accidently ate a peanut and swelled up like a balloon, or maybe a friend who didn't realize he was allergic to shellfish until the middle of the blue crab festival in Maryland. These are extreme examples of food allergies, and though they are some of the most dangerous types of reactions, many of us are having more subtle reactions to foods we eat every day, and they contribute to chronic inflammation and disease.

"Bob" was 60 years old and was very proactive about his health. He was in pretty good shape, although he had always had impaired vision. Bob was careful with his diet, exercised daily, and took a number of supplements including garlic because of its cardioprotective qualities and ability to enhance the immune system. He also enjoyed cooking, and he and his wife both used garlic often when preparing meals. When Bob did his food allergy test, he discovered that he was highly allergic to garlic, of all things. When he cut it out of his diet and supplementation regimen, his vision improved for the first time in 20 years.

There are several types of immune reactions that your body can mount, depending on what the antigen (allergy-causing substance) is, how you come in contact with it, and what kind of antibody you make. An anaphylactic response is a Type I reaction and is caused by IgE antibodies. Foods that cause a Type I reaction are usually obvious because it happens right away. It may not be as serious as the kid with the peanut; it could be just itchy eyes, or bumps on the tongue or lip. Another type of immune response is created using IgG antibodies. This reaction takes much longer to occur. In fact, up to 48 hours can pass before you may start to feel the effects. As you can imagine, this makes the detective work a lot more difficult as the first 48 hours are the most important when trying to solve any mystery—in this case, the mystery being what food is causing the reaction. You probably eat an untold number of foods in a given 48-hour period (yes, we're including the snacks your wife doesn't know about). If you eat these foods that you are allergic to regularly, the re-action adds up as your body is still dealing with inflammation from two days ago. You may unknowingly be adding insult to injury. Fortunately, there are a number of companies who provide testing for food aller-gies. They usually screen for 90 to 100 of the most commonly eaten foods, and the best part is that the IgG antibodies can be tested using just a prick of your finger; you don't even need a blood draw. Please look in the resource section for details about how to access this testing. In our clinical practices, we rou-tinely test for delayed food aller-gens. The symptoms of food allergies can be as complex as the foods that cause them. A couple of the most common include ear infections, eczema, asthma, and diarrhea; the allergies can also contribute to at-tention deficit disorder (ADD), at-tention deficit/hyperactivity disor-der (ADHD), depression, anxiety, headaches and more.

Do you snore? Have you ever been told that you stop breathing in your sleep? If you are a male over the age of 50, there's a 4 percent chance that you are suffering from obstructive sleep apnea (OSA) and if you snore, that number increases to 17 percent. As we covered briefly before, sleep apnea causes a disrup-tion in your sleep, resulting in your body getting little or no restful sleep

"Jeff" is a 46-year-old man with a history of irritable bowel syndrome, chronic lower back pain, and anx-iety. He has been experiencing in-testinal problems since high school. Evaluations by GI specialists indi-cated celiac disease; however, di-etary changes were ineffective in relieving his complaints. We ran the 96 general food-specific IgG panel through USBT. His report showed elevations for yogurt, milk, and peanuts, all of which he had been eating just about every day.

Removal of the moderate and high reactive foods from his diet resulted in about a 30 percent improvement in his IBS symptoms in approxi-mately one week's time. Upon eval-uation at eight weeks, he stated he has seen about an 85 percent im-provement in his GI symptoms with no reoccurring bouts of intestinal distress; he has also experienced sig-nificantly less back pain and sore-ness. He no longer plans his day around finding bathrooms and has felt the most improvement in his symptoms since high school! Jeff was highly allergic to six different foods—by eliminating them from his diet, he has literally changed his life.

(Courtesy of U.S. BioTek Laborato-ries)

despite the fact that you may "think" you are sleeping soundly. The repercussions of sleep apnea range from high blood pressure to chronic daytime sleepiness to testosterone deficiency. The good news is that it is relatively easy to get tested. Your doctor can order a screening test for you. There are many sleep labs across the country that will lend or rent you a machine that will track your oxygen saturation levels throughout the night. When you stop breathing, the percent-age of your tissues that is saturated with oxygen will decrease. From the results

"Clark" is a 42-year-old man who suffered from a gradual decline in health for many years. He was noticing a decreased ability to think clearly, was constantly fatigued, was gaining weight, and had a hard time pinpointing when this change had begun. Eventually, he was treated for sleep apnea, and only after he began sleeping soundly again did he realize what a profound effect his apnea was having on his life. He had been going through the motions of life, but missing out on enjoying it.

Since then, he has been tested and treated for low testosterone as well, which has made him feel even better, but still doesn't compare to the night-and-day difference that treating his apnea made.

In total, he feels a lot more like Superman, not just "Clark."

of this test, you and your doctor can determine if you should continue with a polysomnography (PSG). During a PSG, you will spend the night in the sleep center, and they will record your sleep activity for six to eight hours with an EEG (electroencephalogram), an EMG (eye movement and muscle tone), an ECG (electrocardiogram), and an oxygen saturation machine. These machines will monitor your brain activity, your muscle movements, your heart rate, and your oxygen levels for an extended period of time. The test is non-invasive, doesn't require any needles, and can provide you with important information that could literally save your life.

It is essential to "test not guess," as you move forward with a treatment plan to balance your hormones and restore your body to the youthful way you remember. Testing is just the beginning, but as Confucius said, "A journey of a thousand miles begins with a single step." You've already begun your journey just by reading this book and educating yourself about your body. Gathering more information about your state of health will give you the direction and the motivation to continue on your trip. Not every step along the way will be easy. You are likely to discover that you need to change some portion of your lifestyle that has led to your suboptimal hormone levels and declining health, and changing habits can be difficult. Just keep in mind that the rewards will be great. You can track your progress with additional testing along the way, and celebrate your improvement with youthful energy and vigor.

NOTES

1. Fritz, K.S., A.J. McKean, J.C. Nelson, R.B. Wilcox, "Analog-based free testosterone test results linked to total testosterone concentrations, not free testosterone concentrations," *Clin Chem* (2008) Mar: 54(3):512–6; E-pub 2008 Jan 2. Excerpt from Tietz Textbook of Clinical Chemistry, *3rd Edition*, 1999.

2. Meeran K., A. Hattersley, G. Mould, S.R. Bloom, "Venepuncture causes rapid rise in plasma ACTH." *Br J Clin Pract.* 1993 Sep–Oct;47(5):246–7.

3. Stanczyk, F.Z., R.J. Paulson, S. Roy, "Percutaneous administration of progesterone: blood levels and endometrial protection," *Menopause* (2005) Mar;12(2):232–7.

4. Lee J.R., and V. Hopkins, *Hormone Balance Made Simple: The Essential How-to Guide to Symptoms, Dosage, Timing and More* (Warner Books Publishing, 2006).

5. Holick, M.F., "Vitamin D deficiency," *N Engl J Med* (2007) Jul 19; 357(3):266–81.

6. Brownstein, D., *Iodine. Why You Need It, Why You Can't Live Without It, 2nd Ed* (Medical Alternative Press, 2006).

7. Brownstein, *Iodine*.

CHAPTER 8

Allopathic Approaches to Hormone Therapy: Benefits and Risks

Finally, we have reached the part of the book where we will tell you what you can do about these problems and disease processes that we have been describing all this time. Thanks for bearing with us. We hope you have learned a few things about your body. It's important for you to understand the basic workings of your body so that you can ensure that you are taking the best care of it possible, just as knowing how your vehicle works and being familiar with its various parts and functions allows you to maintain its optimal function and safety. Contrary to popular belief, what you don't know **can** hurt you. Take, for example, the fact that several generations ago it seems like just about everyone in this country smoked. Why not? It was the socially acceptable thing to do and most people had no idea that it was dangerous to their health. The first report linking tobacco smoke to lung disease was actually published in 1836,[1] although most of the dangers of smoking weren't widely recognized by the public until the 1950s and 1960s. We now know that smoking kills more than 400,000 people a year.[2] What's the point here? Well, we'll take every opportunity to tell you that you should not smoke, but we're really trying to tell you that you have the knowledge to understand enough about what is going on in your body to be responsible for your health. Of course you should still see your primary care health provider regularly, but just as you want to be able to talk to your mechanic intelligently about the systems that may go wrong in your car instead of just blindly writing a check for him to fix everything he thinks is wrong, you should understand the basic systems in your body.

This chapter is going to cover some of the more traditional treatments for testosterone insufficiency. In clinical practice, we use some of these treatments often, and some we don't use at all, but they are commonly used by many physicians. For those of you who aren't sure you want to supplement hormones, Chapter 9 will cover some other ways that you may boost your body's own production of testosterone and fight the aging process with some less-direct methods. Depending on your age, this may be the better plan for you. There is no part of this book that is intended to advise you on how to treat your symptoms. We are merely trying to give you an accurate overview of the options out there so that you are well informed and able to communicate with your physician to come up with a treatment plan that is tailored to best fit your needs.

When did people start supplementing testosterone? Well, we have long known about the concept of testosterone and had an idea about the roles it plays in the body. Just as my friends in Louisiana do with their donkeys, there are reports of animals being castrated for domestication purposes going back 6,000 years. It wasn't until 1889 that the 72-year-old French physician Charles-Édouard Brown-Séquard announced to the *Société de Biologie* (Society of Biology) of Paris that he had been injecting himself with an extract made from the testicles of dogs and guinea pigs, and as a result described a radical gain in physical strength as well as mental capacity. Unfortunately, Dr. Brown-Séquard's extract was eventually found to be devoid of any actual androgen hormone, and his experience attributed to placebo. Another 50 years passed until the production of synthetic testosterone was achieved, and Adolf Butenandt and Leopold Ruzicka won the Nobel Prize in Chemistry in 1939 for their synthesis of the male hormone. Once isolated and synthesized, testosterone supplementation began being used for a variety of reasons. One early theory even asserted that sexual preference was related to the ratio of male hormones to female hormones, and testosterone treatments were prescribed as therapy for homosexual men. As you may have guessed, this didn't prove to be successful.[3]

Testosterone was originally synthesized in 1939 and is currently produced in a laboratory setting for clinical use. You have likely heard a lot about bio-identical hormones. In fact, we've probably mentioned that phrase a couple of times in this book. What does that mean exactly? Bio-identical does **not** necessarily mean natural. Bio-identical means that the hormone structure looks exactly like the natural hormone that is found in your body, but says nothing about the way that it is produced. Synthetic hormones are those that have a structure that is different from what you would normally find in your body. Oftentimes, the base hormone is modified to make it more absorbable orally, or to slow down absorption. Synthetic hormones often act on hormone receptors in a similar way to bio-identical hormones and, through this mechanism, have therapeutic value. Unfortunately, they often interact with the body in other ways as well, and, for that reason, are more prone to have adverse side effects. For an example, take a look at the structures of testosterone and estradiol in Figure 8.1.

See how very similar they are. They only differ by one hydrogen atom on the first carbon ring (where there is a double bond between the carbon and oxygen in testosterone and a single bond on the estrogen molecule) and one additional carbon molecule found on testosterone. Now you know how very different the effects that these two molecules have on our bodies, as we've been discussing many of them for over a hundred pages now. Now take a look at the differences

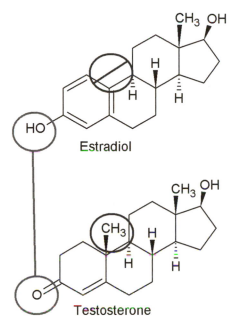

CH₃ OH

Estradiol

CH₃ OH

Testosterone

Figure 8.1 As you can see, have, testosterone and estradiol have remarkably similar structures dispite their very different
actions in the body.

between progesterone and a common progestin (synthetic progesterone) that is
found in many birth control pills. (Figure 8.2)

Of course this book is about men, who are likely not taking birth control
pills, but bear with us for a moment because one of the most common synthetic
hormones used are the progestins found in birth control pills. See how the differences between progesterone and the synthetic norgestimate are significantly
more dramatic than the differences between estrogen and testosterone? Now do
you think that it's possible that the synthetic hormone has a different effect on
the body than its bioidentical counterpart? All hormones (both bio-identical and
synthetic) are created in a lab. Bio-identical hormones are usually created from
a compound found in soy or Mexican yam and modified to look exactly like the
molecule found in our bodies. We use bio-identical hormones almost exclusively
in our practices, but there are occasional reasons why a synthetic hormone may be
necessary. There are many hormones that can be used in a hormone replacement
program, but since this book is primarily about testosterone, let's start by talking
about the various forms of testosterone supplementation available.

TESTOSTERONE

Testosterone can be taken orally; sublingually; injected under your skin or into
your muscle; transmitted through your skin in a cream, a gel, or a patch; implanted
under your skin in little pellets; and even absorbed through your gums. There are

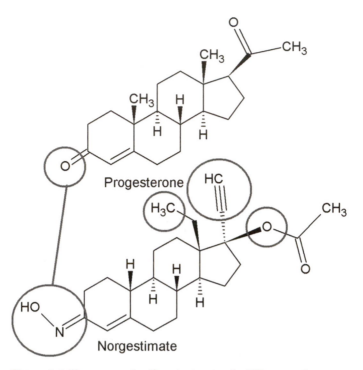

Figure 8.2 There are significant structural differences between bioidentical progesterone and synthetic progestins.

several forms of synthetic testosterone that have been produced in an effort to increase absorption. To make testosterone available as an oral supplement, it must be modified so that we can absorb it.

The first oral testosterone supplements were methylated (a chemical process that makes it more absorbable). Methyltestosterone was one of the original forms of oral testosterone supplementation. Though it is still used today in many supplements including the brand names Methitest®, Android®, Testred®, Virilon®, and Estratest®, there are many warnings against methyltestosterone because of its known toxicity to the liver.[4] We would recommend that you avoid using this form of testosterone. Despite this danger, some sources report that up to one-third of testosterone prescriptions in the United States use these oral preparations. When you consume something orally, it must be absorbed in your intestines regardless of whether it is a vitamin, a protein, a medication, or other substance. Once absorbed through the intestinal wall, it travels into your blood and goes immediately to the liver. In fact, most oral medications experience a significant decrease in bioavailability due to this phenomenon that is called the "first pass" effect. Essentially, a considerable portion of the prescribed amount of the medication is eliminated from the body during its "first pass" through the liver before it even gets to the target tissues. This process adds to the overall burden on the liver. Dosages of medications usually take this into account, and this explains why an oral dose of a medication may be significantly larger than if you were giving the substance under the tongue, in a transdermal cream, patch, or injection.

One oral form of testosterone that is effective, but doesn't add much load to the liver, is a sublingual lozenge or troche (pronounced troh-key fancy word for a lozenge). Testosterone prepared in this fashion has the advantage of bypassing intestinal absorption and, therefore, the "first pass" effect and is relatively easy for patients to do. The hormone is very quickly absorbed when administered in this way, and, therefore, often has to be dosed several times a day because the serum levels

If you are confused about why we keep talking about serum levels, when just a few pages ago we were telling you that our preferred method of testing for and monitoring the therapy of testosterone was through saliva, it's because most of the studies that have been done were done on serum. Like we said, this is the way that the medical community is accustomed to monitoring any body chemistry.

will return to baseline more quickly. Troches can be custom made by a compounding pharmacist in order to customize the dose to meet your individual needs. The custom blending also allows your physician to mix hormones and other compounds together for convenience and cost-effectiveness. The most popular sublingual troches are typically bio-identical, so they don't have any additional structures attached to them and therefore are less likely to have as many adverse side effects. Though a troche is designed to be absorbed into the blood vessels under your tongue, some of it can end up in your saliva and be swallowed. The portion that is swallowed will be absorbed in your intestines and, therefore, does pass through your liver. In theory, this could cause some of the same liver problems that oral testosterone does, but usually the amount that enters your system in this way is minimal. Because the hormone is being absorbed in your mouth, this method of delivery does make it relatively difficult to monitor using saliva testing because the sublingual tissues can be saturated with the hormone. Current guidelines recommend that you stop supplementation 24 to 36 hours prior to giving a saliva sample so that you can accurately monitor hormone therapy.

There is a new product on the market called Striant®,[5] which is a buccal delivery system for testosterone. The buccal area of your mouth is the inside of your cheeks. This delivery system involves a tablet-shaped patch that is affixed to your outer gum (between your lip and your gums). The patch is pressed into place and remains there for approximately eight hours. Striant® has been approved by the FDA and remains relatively uncommon due to its newness, but may have some of the same drawbacks that a sublingual troche does.

We touched on using hormones transdermally when we were discussing various testing methods. Transdermal means "through your skin," and testosterone can be delivered via this mechanism in a patch, a cream, or a gel. Transdermal testosterone is usually bio-identical. Transdermal patches were originally patented in the 1990s and work simply by releasing a fixed amount of the hormone into the skin over time. There are two kinds of testosterone patches; those that are placed on the scrotum, and those that are not. Scrotal patches require that the scrotum be shaved, and the other patches typically go on the lower abdomen or lower back, an area that can also be relatively hairy for many men. All patches have a possibility of inciting an allergic reaction due to the adhesive that comes in contact with the skin. Regardless of its placement, each patch should be changed daily, and among its advantages are the relative ease of use, and the decreased likelihood of contaminating a partner. The primary drawbacks include the skin irritation and the fact that some men have problems with getting the patch to stick and stay on due to excessive hair and sweating. The two primary brands on the market are Androderm® and Testoderm® (generic brand testosterone patches are currently unavailable). For this reason, it can be a relatively expensive option, especially if insurance doesn't help to cover it. Though the dosage of each patch is approximated, there is some variability in absorption.[6]

Transdermal creams and gels tend to be less irritating to the skin than the adhesives and alcohol found in patches. There are many different bases (cream or gel) that you (or your prescribing doctor) can choose from when creating a compounded testosterone supplement, so if one is irritating to the skin, another might not be. Topical creams are custom blended by your local compounding pharmacist, which means that you have infinite variability with dosage. Like the troche, since these creams are made for each patient individually, they can be blended with other hormones as well. As you can imagine, it's much easier to have all of your hormone supplements in one place. It gives you less to remember, less to carry around, etc. The creams are typically less expensive than many of the other routes of administration; however, some men do find that they have mild difficulty with application. The sites on your body where you rub the cream need to be areas where your skin is relatively thin. The inner arms, backs of the knees, tops of the feet, and occasionally upper chest work pretty well for most men. If you rub the cream into an area where there is a lot of fat, the hormone is absorbed into the fat and a reservoir is created. This makes it much more difficult to monitor how much hormone you are getting since the fat tissues will sometimes hold on to the hormones, and then release it slowly back into the system. Another drawback to topical creams is the possibility of transferring some of the cream to someone that you have close physical contact with. After the cream is applied, it's important that you thoroughly wash your hands. While we prefer in our clinical practice to use creams and gels that are compounded (and, therefore, custom blended for our patients), there are some manufactured topical testosterone products on the market. AndroGel®, for example, is a very popular product. In fact, they claim that it's the number one testosterone replacement product on the market. AndroGel® is a 1 percent solution, and it comes in either 2.5 g or 5 g packets or a pump that delivers 1.25 g with each pump. A 1 percent mixture means that there is 10 mg of testosterone in each gram of gel, and, therefore, a 2.5 g dose actually delivers 25 mg of testosterone to the skin.[7]

Testosterone injections may remind you of certain major league ballplayers and their trainers, but, in fact, this is a popular method of delivery, especially in Europe. The testosterone must be esterified, which improves the solubility of the hormone in oil and permits a longer-lasting effect in the body. This is done to prevent the user from having to inject every day. The esterification process is a chemical process where the molecule is modified to allow it to be longer acting. There are several possible products available on the market. In the past, testosterone cypionate, testosterone propionate, and testosterone undecanoate were injected every two weeks. At two-week intervals, the amount that must be injected causes the levels in the body to be much higher than "normal" in the beginning, and they become very low again at the end of the two weeks. For this reason, injection of a smaller amount once a week is recommended to keep testosterone levels more even. Allowing the testosterone levels to be too high, even for just a few days, causes more side effects including more aromatization to estradiol and more of an increase in red blood cell density, all of which we want to avoid.

Yet another delivery method for testosterone is pellets that are compounded by the pharmacist and implanted into the tissues just below the skin of the lower abdominal wall. This requires a minor incision at the implantation site, but the procedure only has to be done every four to six months. The pellets provide adequate hormone release and there is minimal elevation of estradiol and DHT. Of course, there are occasional problems at the site of implantation, and many people just plain don't like the idea of implanting something under their skin. Another drawback to both the implantations and the injections is the fact that once the substance is in your body, it can't be readily removed so dosage adjustments are difficult. With oral or transdermal administration, it is easier to modify the dose based on symptoms.

Although we use testosterone as a very successful treatment for many of our patients, please remember that there can be some significant side effects if the therapy isn't monitored properly, and this isn't necessarily a treatment for everyone. Just to reiterate, your PSA levels should be checked **prior** to starting therapy, because although testosterone doesn't cause prostate cancer, it can stimulate the cancer to grow more quickly if it already exists. We would not recommend that you supplement your body with testosterone if you have prostate or breast cancer. Yes, we said breast cancer. Though it's not nearly as common in men as it is with women (for obvious reasons), men can and do get breast cancer. If you know that you have impaired kidney or liver functions, you should be extra careful about any substance you put in your body as your liver is responsible for clearing your body of toxins and chemicals, both those that your body produces as well as the ones you are exposed to from outside sources. Testosterone supplementation will likely cause your testicles to shrink in size somewhat, and will lower your sperm count. So again, a reminder, if you have a need or desire to be fertile, you may want to take a different approach.

If you do decide to pursue a treatment plan that includes supplementation with testosterone, you should give yourself several months of treatment before you judge whether or not it is working. Many people notice a difference almost immediately, yet for others the changes are more subtle. Hormone treatment

Route of Administration	Pros	Cons
Oral	• Conventional, most people are used to taking medications this way	• Toxic to the liver • Lose much of the dose to the first pass effect
Sublingual (Troche)	• Easy to use • Compounded, so able to custom blend for individual • Absorbs quickly	• Difficult to monitor progress with salivary hormone test • Some hormone is swallowed • Often needed to be administered at least twice a day for optimal effect
Transdermal Patch	• Easy to use • Not transferred to family members • Evenly administered dose	• Skin irritation • Difficult with hair or sweat • Expensive
Transdermal Cream	• Custom compounded • Variety of creams or gels to choose from to eliminate allergies • Less expensive	• Possibility of contaminating family member • Possibility of allergic skin reaction
Injectable	• Only has to be done once a week • Evenly administered dose	• Involves needles • Occasional inflammation at injection site • Reduced ability to alter dose
Implantable	• Very even physiologic dose • No elevation of DHT or estradiol	• Requires a minor procedure • No flexibility with dosage

Table 8.1 The Pros and Cons of the various forms of testosterone supplementation.

isn't a panacea. Though we have covered many symptoms that often improve for people when they balance their hormones, there is no guarantee that everything will be perfect. Sorry. Re-testing to monitor therapy should be at least every three months until you have established a dosage and regimen that consistently maintains your hormones at optimal levels. Don't monitor therapy by symptoms alone! PSA levels should also be monitored every three months initially. The enzymatic pathways in the body that turn testosterone into estrogen and DHT work at different rates in many different people, so a dosage that works for you may not work for your brother or your neighbor. What happens if you fall into the category of men who aromatize (that's the conversion of testosterone to estrogen) more readily than others? There are a couple of things you can do: first of all, make an effort to lose weight as the aromatase is most active in adipose (fat) cells, second, you can often use or take a substance that acts as an aromatase inhibitor, which means that it blocks the action of that enzyme and third, you can enhance your body's ability to metabolize and get rid of estrogens.

Aromatase inhibitors are a classification of drugs that are used for many different purposes. They are perhaps most commonly found in the treatment of breast and ovarian cancer, in an effort to further reduce the presence of estrogen in women whose tumors have been shown to have receptors for (and be stimulated by) estrogen. So while the *Oprah* crowd may be familiar with aromatase inhibitors, the other group that frequently uses them is bodybuilders. For the reasons we described when we were discussing the effects of excess testosterone, many bodybuilders and athletes who supplement androgen hormones find that they must take an aromatase inhibitor as well to prevent gynecomastia (the formation of breast tissue). What are these aromatase inhibitors? Well, there are a number of pharmaceuticals including anastrozole (Arimidex®, Android®); letrozole (Femara®, Android®); and exemestane (Aromasin®, Android®); and more. Some natural substances that have been shown to have aromatase inhibitory properties include chrysin (from passiflora), apigenin (from chamomile), genistein, and diadzein (from soy). These compounds will be covered in more detail in our next chapter, but we wanted to briefly mention the fact that there are several options beyond pharmaceuticals.

If aromatizing to estrogen isn't your problem, but you seem to convert testosterone to DHT, then there are similar compounds that disrupt the enzyme 5-alpha reductase that converts testosterone into the more potent DHT. Finasteride (marketed as Proscar®, Android®, Propecia®, Android®, and others) is a synthetic compound that has been shown to disturb this pathway. These drugs are marketed for hair loss and to treat prostate enlargement, because the enzyme 5-alpha reductase is most active in prostate cells and hair follicles and the DHT stimulates proliferation of the prostate tissue and destruction of hair follicles. Be warned, there are some significant side effects with this compound, including severe birth defects if a pregnant woman is exposed to it. Some natural substances that have a similar action are saw palmetto, plant sterols, and others that will be covered in the chapter on natural treatments.

So, what if you are one of the younger men reading this book? Maybe you don't have any kids yet, or still want to have a few more, and you have heeded the warning that supplementation with testosterone can lower your sperm count. If you still need your sperm to swim like Michael Phelps, one option is to consult with your doctor about the use of human chorionic gonadotropin (HCG). HCG is a protein that is produced by pregnant women and is the substance that is measured in pregnancy tests. Home pregnancy tests turn blue to indicate that there is presence of HCG in the urine. HCG is also what is measured quantitatively in blood to confirm pregnancy for many women. "So what", you're thinking. Don't worry. We are not going to take this equality with healthcare thing so far as to suggest that men attempt to become pregnant! Actually, one whole subunit (component) of HCG is identical to luteinizing hormone (LH), which you may remember is the hormone that stimulates the Leydig cells to produce testosterone. In men who want to retain their fertility and know that they don't have Leydig cell failure, HCG treatment may stimulate the Leydig cells in the same way that LH does.[8] For this reason, HCG is used by some physicians when treating younger men for testosterone deficiency and when treating men with fertility problems. It's also given in a cycle with testosterone to maintain normal testicle size and tone with many patients. HCG has been suggested by many to be a potent weight-loss aid and is marketed as such in many books and on many Web sites. Dr. A.T.W. Simeons first began writing about the relationship between HCG and weight loss.[9] He found that when combined with a very low calorie diet (500 calories/day) the patients using HCG were less hungry, less irritable, and had fewer headaches. Though it has been purported as a treatment for obesity for almost 50 years, the evidence that it works as a weight-loss product are mixed. It's likely that the weight loss that many people report is caused by the stimulation of testosterone, and through this mechanism, their bodies are more anabolic. At any rate, this is a product that requires that you work closely with a physician who knows what he or she is doing.

We touched on the topic of growth hormone when we were discussing testing IGF-1, or insulin-like growth factor, which is a reflection of growth hormone levels. Your natural production of growth hormone is stimulated by the hypothalamic-pituitary axis like most of the other hormones we have discussed. The use of growth hormones as a supplement is a controversial topic. Of course, they have been used for many years to treat growth hormone deficiency and prevent dwarfism, but the use of HGH as an anti-aging treatment remains cutting edge. There are clearly many benefits, and the proponents of this treatment claim that it prevents or reverses aging; rejuvenates the immune system; reverses heart failure; builds bones; improves energy, mood, and sleep quality; enhances sexual function; controls obesity; and more. Sounds pretty good, doesn't it? The opponents of the therapy warn that HGH supplementation can cause carpal tunnel syndrome, high blood pressure, osteoporosis, impotence, heat intolerance, insulin resistance, headaches, fluid retention, and gynecomastia. However, these were the effects of dosing to achieve higher than physiologic levels. There may be a link to breast and prostate cancer as well. Aside from the possible risks, the treatment is extremely expensive and relatively difficult to obtain legally. A full year's worth of treatment could cost as much as $30,000. New brands of the hormone may lower the cost to as much as $3,000 per year, but this is still relatively expensive for many people, especially compared with the many natural ways to boost your body's production of growth hormone.

There are some other therapies that you may have heard of; androstenedione for example, is an immediate precursor to testosterone in the hormone pathways. It was once available over the counter as a dietary supplement and will increase testosterone levels. [10] "Andro," as it is commonly called, is perhaps best known for its use by Mark McGuire when he first broke Babe Ruth's single-season home run record in 1998. Since that time, it has been banned by the World Anti-Doping Agency as well as Major League Baseball and was banned by the FDA in 2004. Other precursor supplements such as this **can** feed into the testosterone pathway, but that doesn't mean that all of them will, and the process isn't very precise. Just as we talked about how different people have varying efficiencies of their aromatase enzymes, the conversion pathways of all of these hormones can vary significantly. DHEA is the androgen hormone that is produced by the adrenal glands. Your body's production of DHEA will decline significantly with age (we call this adrenopause). DHEA plays a role in stress response and stress management, but also significantly affects your physiology through its conversion to either estrogen or testosterone. Many people report that DHEA supplementation significantly improves their quality of life and overall sense of well-being. It is being studied in the treatment of many diseases including Alzheimer's and adrenal fatigue. Though DHEA is available over the counter, its use should really be supervised by a physician and monitored with salivary hormone levels to ensure that the DHEA isn't feeding the estrogen pathway and driving estrogen levels up or adversely affecting testosterone levels.

While we're on the subject of testosterone and other hormone supplementation, we should probably at least mention that one of the areas where we see these hormones used therapeutically the most is not in clinics and hospitals, but in gyms and training facilities. The use of steroids is not just the stuff of after-school specials. There are thousands of men, women, boys, and girls out there who are using a wide assortment of hormones to alter their bodies. If you've never been involved in or exposed to this world, you should know that it is extensive and not particularly clandestine. Spend a few minutes on the Internet, and you can learn all about the "underground world" of illegal steroids. Furthermore, it's not just the world of bodybuilding where you see anabolic steroids being used; these substances are ubiquitous among athletes at many levels. A study done in 1989 surveyed a little over 1,000 high-school students and found that 5 percent of males and 1.4 percent of females reported using anabolic steroids.[11] Another study in 2006, this time looking in the reasons why people use anabolic steroids, found that of the 500 people surveyed, 78 percent of them weren't even doing it for performance-enhancing reasons. Their motivations were purely cosmetic.[12] While we have advocated repeatedly that you become aware and educated about your health, and we want you to be empowered, we do not recommend that you use anabolic steroids for cosmetic or any other purpose. The testosterone supplementation that we practice and are promoting is responsible, bio-identical replacement of your hormones that does not exceed healthy physiologic doses.

Testosterone isn't the only hormone that we recommend to men. Progesterone plays a very important role in protecting your prostate from any growth, benign or otherwise. Progesterone is the "other female hormone" that helps to balance the proliferative effects of estrogen. Remember, the aging hormone picture isn't purely about declining testosterone; you also experience increasing estrogen levels. Men don't need the same amount of progesterone in their bodies as women do, but supplementing a little will provide your breast tissue and prostate with some extra protection. We included this hormone in the allopathic approaches chapter because we are discussing the other hormones; however, it is relatively uncommon to see conventional doctors prescribe progesterone for men and, in fact, many of them overlook this hormone even with women.

If you have marked low cortisol levels, especially if your morning cortisol is low, you may want to consider the short-term use of low doses of cortisol until the underlying cause of the adrenal insufficiency (often called adrenal burnout) is addressed. Cortisol is the name of the hormone that your body produces, and hydrocortisone is the name of the synthetic version. At high levels, cortisol can suppress the immune system, suppress testosterone production, and encourage the body to store fat and manufacture glucose much like the stress response we profiled a few chapters ago. For this reason, we use doses that are within physiologic ranges, meaning that they won't stimulate the reactions that a stress response surge of cortisol or a pharmacologic dose of synthetic cortisol will. Cortisol doses of less than 20 mg/day can give your body some relief from adrenal fatigue and make you feel remarkably different. Cortisol should be given in divided doses, and should mimic the natural diurnal pattern, with the greatest amount given in the morning. Unlike your testicles and testosterone production, the adrenal glands are capable of manufacturing adequate amounts of cortisol until very late in life if they are treated well and given proper nourishment. Unfortunately, many of us abuse our adrenal system with our high stress lifestyles and inadequate rest and relaxation. We'll go over this a little more when we get to the prevention portion of the book, which we've chosen to place toward the end. Although it would be logical to start with prevention, unfortunately only hindsight is 20/20 and we don't tend to think about prevention until we have been through some measure of trouble to begin with. We want to first make it clear what all of the consequences could be if you aren't proactive about your health.

NOTES

1. Samuel Green, *New England Almanack and Farmer's Friend* (1836).

2. Centers for Disease Control and Prevention. Cigarette smoking-attributable mortality and years of potential life lost—United States, 1990. *Morbidity and Mortality Weekly Report* [serial online]. 1993;42(33):645–649. Available from: http://www.cdc.gov/mmwr/preview/mmwrhtml/00021441.htm.

3. Freeman, E.R., D.A. Bloom, E.J. McGuire, "A brief history of testosterone," *J Urol*, 165:371, 2001.

4. Westaby, D., S.J. Ogle, F.J. Paradinas, J.B. Randell, I.M. Murray-Lyon, "Liver damage from long-term methyltestosterone," *Lancet* (1977) Aug 6;2(8032):262–3.

5. Wang, C., R. Swerdloff, M. Kipnes, A.M. Matsumoto, A.S. Dobs, G. Cunningham, L. Katznelson, T.J. Weber, T.C. Friedman, P. Snyder, H.L. Levine, "New testosterone buccal system (Striant®, Android®) delivers physiological testosterone levels: pharmacokinetics study in hypogonadal men," J Clin Endocrinol Metab (2004) Aug;89(8):3821–9.

6. www.rxlist.com.

7. www.androgel.com.

8. Liu, P.Y., S.M. Wishart, D.J. Handelsman, "A double-blind, placebo-controlled, randomized clinical trial of recombinant human chorionic gonadotropin on muscle srength and physical function and activity in older men with partial age-related androgen deficiency," *J Clin Endocrinol Metab* (2002) July;87(7):3125–3135.

9. Simmeions, A.T.W., *Pounds and Inches: A New Approach to Obesity*; http://www.hcgdietinfo.com/HCG_Diet_Dr_Simeons_Manuscript.htm.

10. Leder, B.Z., D.H. Catlin, C. Longcope, B. Ahrens, D.A. Shoenfeld, J.S. Finkelstein. "Metabolism of orally administered androstenedione in young men," *J Clin Endocrin & Metab*:86(8):3654–3658.

11. Windsor, R. and D. Dumitru, "Prevalence of anabolic steroid use by male and female adolescents," *Med Sci Sports Exerc* (1989): Oct;21(5):494–7.

12. Parkinson, A.B. and N.A. Evans, "Anabolic androgenic steroids: a survey of 500 users," *Med Sci Sports Exerc* (2006) Apr;38(4):644–51.

CHAPTER 9

Natural Medicine Approaches to Hormone Therapy

As physicians who practice natural medicine, we are both excited and cautious of the growing interest in natural therapies. It's an exciting field and it's an exciting time, as more and more Americans are questioning the mediocre status quo of heath care they have been receiving over the years and are beginning to think outside the box and look at all of their options. The fact is that health care has become a disease management system, and there is no time in history where

> It's far more important to know what person the disease has than what disease the person has.—Hippocrates

there have been more people suffering from ailments due to overindulgences, premature aging, and chronic diseases. We are very excited to be in a position to educate people about their bodies, their health, and their diverse choices. At the same time, we are wary of popular opinion that says if a treatment or therapy is "natural," then it must be safe. There are many, many compounds in nature that can have profound effects on your body, both positively and negatively. In fact, some of the most powerful pharmaceuticals are created from herbal constituents. Did you know that approximately 25 percent of commonly prescribed "prescription drugs" have natural origins?

You have likely heard of the humble beginnings of penicillin—accidentally discovered in a mold. Opioid derivatives such as hydrocodone, oxycodone, and codeine come from the poppy plant. Digitalis, a common heart medication, comes from foxglove. Aspirin originally came from the white willow tree. Even several chemotherapy drugs—Vinicristine from periwinkle and Taxol® from the Yew tree—are derived from nature. Now, we have encouraged you throughout this book to feel empowered in regards to your health, and we mean it. We're

The Principles of Naturopathic Medicine

The healing power of nature—Your body has an innate ability to heal itself.

Identify and treat the cause—Wellness cannot be restored unless the underlying cause is identified and eliminated.

First do no harm—Like the Hippocratic oath states, the physician shouldn't employ any therapies that cause harm or discomfort to the patient.

Treat the whole person—All aspects of an organism are connected; physical, emotional, spiritual, and mental wellness are necessary for optimal health.

Doctor as teacher—The role of the doctor is not to "fix" the problem, but to educate and empower the patient to be responsible for their well-being.

Prevention—The best way to treat a disease is to avoid getting it at all.

not going back now and telling you that you should rely solely on what your doctor tells you. We are merely asserting that it's important to do your research and learn about any therapy you begin, whether it is something prescribed by your trusted family doctor, something that the grocery store clerk suggested, or you read about it in a book (including this book), or on the Web. We feel that it's best to work with your doctors and make sure that they are all informed about all substances that you are using as it will give them the necessary information to be in the best position to recommend what is best for you. It's not only important to know what the effects of any herb, supplement, or medication you may be taking will be, but you must also look at the way that they will impact each other. I (C. Meletis) have written or coauthored four books that address the topic of interactions between natural medicines and herbs. Some of these interactions can be very powerful. For example, St. John's wort, an herb used for mild depression and antiviral properties, can increase the body's ability to clear medications, so it can decrease the amount of your prescription medication, often to levels below therapeutic value.

There are many times in medicine where the line is blurred between natural therapies and allopathic or conventional treatments. Before we go into specific treatments, we want to explain that we believe that the therapy used or the medication prescribed does not necessarily define the philosophy behind it. For example, we are often asked what exactly a "naturopathic physician" is or does. This question is especially common when we travel to one of the states where we aren't licensed as primary care providers, as we are in our home state of Oregon. (There are many states whose laws don't yet define a scope of practice for natural physicians, and, therefore, do not offer a license.) Many people venture that the primary difference between an ND and an MD would be prescriptions; an MD gives pharmaceuticals and performs surgery, while an ND suggests herbs or nutritional supplements. While these statements may be true a large percentage of the time, they do not define the core difference between the two. In Oregon and several other states, naturopathic physicians can write prescriptions for a wide variety of pharmaceuticals including controlled substances that require a DEA number. We frequently prescribe medications from a pharmacy, but do so in accordance with the philosophy that the therapy is treating the cause of the problem and not just masking a symptom. There are six principles of naturopathic medicine, and this is where you truly find the philosophical difference with a natural approach to your health. **How** you employ an herb or a pharmaceutical in a healing process is more important than **what** therapy you use. Of course, every decision should be based on what is best for the patient, and any personal philosophies or biases regarding pharmaceuticals or natural therapies should be put aside to give the patient the best care possible.

The word "natural" can have several different meanings depending on how you look at it. Hormone replacement therapy is a perfect example of an area where there may be a discrepancy. As we discussed in the last chapter, we frequently use bio-identical hormones. These hormones are formulated to be identical to the compounds found in your body, so their actions on your tissues are "natural" or similar to the actions of nature. They are created in a lab from natural sources, usually soy or yam. Does this make them natural because the starting material comes from nature or synthetic even though they are man-made creations? The most commonly prescribed hormone worldwide is Premarin®: it's been given to menopausal women all over the world for more than 50 years. Premarin® is a conjugated estrogen product made from the urine of pregnant mares. (This is where it gets its name: **Pregnant-mares-urine** = Premarin®.) Well, that seems pretty natural, doesn't it? Horse urine sounds like the kind of thing you would expect to hear used by some remote tribe in the Amazon. The truth is that Premarin® couldn't be more mainstream; it is one of the most often prescribed pharmaceuticals and, unfortunately, we are discovering that it has many dangerous side effects in the body. It turns out that though these compounds are more or less taken directly from nature, the actions that they have in our bodies are not very "natural" because they don't look like the endogenous hormones that humans produce—they look like the hormones and byproducts of hormones that pregnant horses produce. So what is "natural" to you?

To some extremists, employing any medicine or therapy is not "natural." To many of these groups of people, the "natural" way is whatever your body is capable of without assistance. Of course, many of these people find themselves facing lawsuits when they don't provide their children with an adequate standard of care, as most of modern society would consider their behavior neglectful. There are many out there who would argue that any hormone replacement therapy or anti-aging therapy is not "natural" as we are supposed to age. On the other end of the spectrum, there are people out there who employ so many substances, procedures, and surgeries that they can completely lose sight of what their bodies would look like "naturally." Does this bring to mind a certain pop star whose face has changed so much over time that he doesn't even resemble the child star he once was? Remember the old slogan "Better living through chemistry?"

This DuPontad slogan was dropped decades ago, as public opinion generally switched from admiring technology and chemicals to fearing the repercussions of the many synthetic compounds we were introducing into our world. Each of you reading this book is likely to have a slightly different view or opinion on what you believe is "natural" and what level of medical and technological intervention is acceptable in our lives. Each situation and case must be weighed individually, for blanket policies may result in the kind of inflexibility that prevents loving parents from providing their children with the basic intervention needed to save their lives. What do we advocate, you ask? As we covered a few chapters ago, we suggest you avoid chemicals and pharmaceuticals that are known to have adverse affects on your body, and be wary and judicious with the use of new substances for which you may not know all of the repercussions yet. We also believe that you should do whatever is in your power to enhance the quality of your life and that the key to this is preventing disease processes, proactively providing your body with the building blocks and nutrients it needs, and maintaining healthy hormone levels.

We don't need to cover bio-identical hormones again in this chapter as we just went over them. Suffice it to say that they probably belong in both categories and the use of bio-identical compounds to restore healthy physiological (normal) levels of hormone is a safe and **natural** approach to health. The use of any of these substances, bio-identical or otherwise, to create falsely high levels of these hormones is **artificial** and dangerous. So what else can you do to enhance your body's production of testosterone? There are a number of nutritional supplements that can stimulate overall testosterone production, as well as optimize your level of free testosterone. Still another group of compounds helps to protect the prostate, enhance libido, or stimulate growth hormone production.

HERBAL SUPPLEMENTS

Longjack, or *Eurycoma longifolia*, is a shrub found in Southeast Asia that has been used for centuries to enhance male prowess. The plant is also called Tongkat Ali, or Pasak Bumi, in some circles and, like many herbs, the history of its use greatly precedes its known mechanism of action. Recent studies have shown that *Eurycoma longifolia* extract has androgenic effects in animal studies.[1] There have been some reports of the extract increasing men's free testosterone levels 50 to 300 percent over a six-month period; however, thorough clinical trials have not been published. Of course, as with any plant you will likely see dosages include the extract ratio. This number tells you how many grams of the whole plant were used to make one gram of the extract and is often noted as a ratio (XX whole plant: XX extract). It appears from the empirical data that an extract of *Eurycoma longifolia* should be at least (20:1) and dosages should be approximately 150 to 250 mg/day. Extracts from the *Eurycoma* plant have been found to have anti-malarial, antipyretic (fever reducing), and antitumor qualities. Further research will likely elucidate more specific information, and it's important to remind you that most of the formal studies on this herb have been done on rats, so its safety hasn't been completely established.

This is a good time to talk about quality of supplements. Please also see our resource section in the back of the book for a list of some reputable companies that we know to have good manufacturing processes and high standardization. There is a book called a *Comparative Guide to Nutritional Supplements* by Lyle MacWilliams that has done independent studies on a large number of nutritional products out there. They indicate that only 1 percent of supplements tested earned a score of 90 percent or better. That means of the 1,000 supplements selected for testing, only 10 were graded with an "A." If you purchase a low-quality supplement, you have no way of knowing if you are actually getting enough of the active ingredient to provide you with symptom relief. At the end of the day, what is more expensive, to take something that doesn't work, or to spend the extra money to purchase a supplement that has been standardized and independently assayed?

Tribulus terrestris is another botanical, traditionally used in ayurvedic medicine, that has shown encouraging results in recent studies. The active constituent of Tribulus is an extract called protodioscin and has been shown to increase testosterone levels in studies done on rats and primates. These studies indicate a significant increase in testosterone and DHEA levels with an intravenous dose of 7.5 mg/kg of bodyweight.[2] *Tribulus* is also known as puncture vine and has been used historically as a "male tonic" for

Categories of Nutritional Supplements Men's Health:

Testosterone boosting:

- *Eurycoma longifolia* (longjack)
- *Eucommia ulmoides* (gutta percha bark)
- *Tribulus terrestris*
- *Epimedium grandiflorum* (horny goat weed)

SHBG binding:

- *Urtica dioica* (stinging nettles)

Aromatase inhibitors:

- Chrysin
- Luteolin
- Apigenin

5-alpha reductase inhibitors:

- *Serenoa repens* (saw palmetto)
- Beta-sitosterol
- *Lepedium meyenii* (Maca)
- Myricetin

Other prostate protective supplements:

- *Pygeum africanum*
- Lycopene
- Zinc
- Selenium
- DIM (diindolylmethane)
- Vitamin D

Libido enhancers:

- *Muira puama*
- *Panax ginseng*

Note: These statements have not be evaluated by the Food and Drug Administration and are not intended to diagnose, treat, cure or prevent any disease.

treating impotence. *Tribulus* is likely to be the subject of many ongoing studies in years to come, as these first studies are optimistic. This herb is expected to become a major player in the future treatment of low androgen levels in men as well as women. An adequate dosage would be approximately 250 mg/day. As with many natural supplements, the long-term safety has not been well studied, but *Tribulus* has been safely used in studies for up to eight weeks.

Horny goat weed (or *Epimedium grandiflorum*) doesn't just **sound** like something that would help with sexual function. There are a number of constituents found in horny goat weed that may play a role in male enhancement. In fact, it's one of the most popular products that you will find in the infomercials for erectile dysfunction products. There are several flavonoids including apigenin and luteolin that have been shown to be aromatase inhibitors, some glycosides that may stimulate testosterone production,[3] and another constituent that may inhibit the same enzyme that Viagra® blocks. In addition, *Epimedium* may block calcium channels, preventing vasoconstriction and inducing vasodilation, which would increase blood flow to the penis (as well as other parts of the body). This is certainly an herb that requires more research. This plant is a good example of one that contains many compounds that we are able to isolate and study independently. While this gives us the opportunity to learn more about each part of the plant, to study it in the conventional "double-blind, placebo controlled" style, and sometimes enables us to create specialized medicines for specific conditions, it also removes some of the "natural" synergy of the plant. There we go with the "natural" stuff again, but there are a lot of people who believe that there is a reason why a plant would contain so many different compounds that act in different ways. This sometimes creates a balance that we are unable to recreate with isolated substances. Epimedium, for example, has some phytoestrogen or estrogen-like compounds in it, but also contains several aromatase inhibiting substances that would help to prevent testosterone from being converted to estrogen and create an overall hormonal imbalance. This is sometimes referred to as the "wisdom" of the plant and is a good reason to use whole plant extracts. As with all things, there are multiple sides to this discussion, and the opponents would argue that it's beneficial to be able to be exact in our therapies, without the added influence of additional substances. You are likely to have your own opinion about this subject and that may be based on your experience or exposure to botanical medicines verses. pharmaceuticals.

As we profiled earlier in this book, much of the problem with waning testosterone levels is the decreasing percentage that is **bioavailable**, which is a phenomenon that is largely due to the increase in SHBG levels that occur with aging. The SHBG (sex hormone binding globulin, in case you forgot) binds up more of the testosterone, which leaves even less of it to act on the tissues. *Urtica dioica*, also known as stinging nettle root extract, is an herbal supplement that binds to SHBG and ties it up,[4] preventing it from binding the testosterone. Specifically, it is a lignan called 3,4-divanillyltetrahydrofuran that binds to SHBG. Stinging nettles is a relatively safe supplement and has been in studies for up to six months of use; however, there are a number of people who find that they have an allergic reaction to nettles. You can have an allergic reaction to almost anything that you put into your body, and if you ever notice an adverse reaction, especially when you have recently begun a new supplementation regimen, you should discontinue what you are taking and then add things back in one at a time to see what is causing the problem, and certainly consult your doctor. Recommended dosage of *uttica dioica* is approximately 120 mg twice daily.

The conversion of testosterone to estrogen causes several problems for men. The first is a deficit in testosterone. When a significant portion of the testosterone that your body is producing is being turned into estrogen instead of acting on the androgen receptors, it will exacerbate a situation where there are already sub-optimal testosterone levels. In fact, even if your body is producing an adequate amount of testosterone, if you are aromatizing much of it to estrogen, then you will end up with a shortage overall. Remember that the aromatase enzyme (the enzyme that converts testosterone to estrogen) is most active in fat tissue. It's not just important to minimize the conversion of testosterone to estrogen because you need the testosterone, but the estrogen will also cause your prostate cells to grow, causing a number of urinary symptoms and will possibly lead to a condition called benign prostatic hypertrophy and even prostate cancer. We mentioned the role of the aromatase enzyme in the last chapter and listed some of the pharmaceuticals that block aromatization. There are also a number of compounds that we find in nutritional supplements that act as aromatase inhibitors. Chrysin is a flavonoid that occurs in several different plants but is most commonly found in passionflower and some geranium species.[5] There are some concerns as to how well chrysin is absorbed into the body because most of the studies proving its efficacy have only been done in the lab. Luteolin and its cousin apigenin are flavonoids with similar anti-aromatase properties,[6] but may be better absorbed than chrysin.[7] As with so many nutritional supplements, we still have so much to learn about these compounds and their mechanisms of action. Dosage of chrysin when taken orally should be 250 to 300 mg/day, and it can be compounded in with topical hormones, but the creams appear to become gritty at dosages over 50 mg/mL. Luteolin dosages of 40 mg/day are often sufficient.

Estrogen plays a large role in prostate disease, causing proliferation of tissues along with DHT (dihydrotestosterone). The enzyme that converts testosterone into DHT is called 5-alpha reductase, and its activity can be blocked by plant sterols such as beta-sitosterol and compounds myricetin and saw palmetto. If you recognize any of these herbs that we have listed so far, it is likely saw palmetto. It's a very popular product marketed for men's health. Saw palmetto is also known as *Serenoa repens* and is one of the first lines of treatment for prostate problems and male baldness. Both actions are through the inhibition of the 5-alpha reductase enzyme.[8] Saw palmetto has been marketed in France since 1982 under the name Permixon®, and is used throughout Europe. A multicenter study in Europe found that twice-daily dosing of 120 mg of saw palmetto was as effective as finasteride (the pharmaceutical we know as Proscar®), but didn't have the side effect of loss of libido.[9] In the United States, saw palmetto is found in health food stores in a variety of products usually targeted at the prostate.

Beta-sitosterol is a plant sterol. Plant sterols cholesterols that come from plants, and we find beta-sitosterol in a number of places including Maca (*Lepedium meyenii*).[10] Plant sterols can have a number of positive effects on the body including lowering cholesterol levels because of their competition for absorption.[11] In the prostate, beta-sitosterol has been shown to have 5-alpha reductase blocking activity[12] similar to the mechanism of action for saw palmetto.

Myricitin[13] is a flavonoid that comes from grape skins, and it works to block the enzyme to prevent conversion of testosterone to DHT as well. Finally, one additional inhibitor of 5-alpha reductase is **progesterone**. We discussed the protective effects of progesterone during the last chapter when we were discussing hormone supplementation, but it's worth mentioning again that not only does it balance the proliferative effects of estrogen on the prostate, but it also inhibits testosterone's conversion to DHT.[14] In addition, progesterone stimulates the activity of a protective gene that promotes the healthy demise of cells in the prostate and therefore helps to control cellular overgrowth.[15]

Pygeum africanum is an extract from the bark of an evergreen tree from Africa and has been shown to have tremendous antiproliferative effect in the cells of the prostate, though not due to the mechanisms listed above.[16] If you are suffering from symptoms of an enlarged prostate—increased urinary frequency, dribbling or split stream, or other urinary problems—you should consider a number of these therapies to control the growth of your prostate while also optimizing your hormone levels. Standard dosing for Pygeum would be between 75 and 200 mg daily in one or divided doses.

Along with the substances that have been studied for measurable increases in testosterone production and treatment for prostate issues, there are a number of compounds that have been used historically to enhance libido and help men attain and sustain an erection. With many of these substances, we don't know exactly which extract of the plant is responsible for the reported medicinal properties. Of course, we need many more studies on these herbs, especially when we have empirical evidence that they are having an effect. *Muira puama*, for example, is also called potency wood and has been used in the Amazon region for treating sexual debility and baldness. When analyzed, potency wood was found to be rich in beta-sitosterol and other plant sterols, essential fatty acids, and an alkaloid called muirapuamine.[17] Some preliminary trials found that up to 85 percent of test subjects experienced an enhanced libido and 90 percent experienced improved ability to maintain an erection.[18] From this study, it seems that this herb clearly deserves more study, so stay tuned. You may hear more about this herb in the future. Dosage of *Muira puama* should be approximately 500 mg of extract three times a day.

Many "male enhancement" products employ herbs that are simply known to increase blood flow or to relax blood vessels in the body. For the most part, these supplements are going to address difficulties with erectile dysfunction, but not the overall reduction in testosterone. *Panax ginseng* is also called Korean, Chinese, or Asian ginseng, but is not to be confused with American or Siberian ginseng, for it is a different plant. *Panax ginseng* has been shown to relax smooth muscle by increasing nitric oxide production, which increases circulation and relaxes the corpus cavernosal smooth muscle.[19] One human study determined that patients given *Panax ginseng* noticed an improvement in penile rigidity, girth, duration of erection, and improved libido compared to placebo groups.[20]

Speaking of "male enhancement" products, you have probably noticed that these products are flooding the market. From late-night infomercials to unsolicited e-mails, you are constantly barraged with information on how you can make your penis longer, bigger, and harder. Most of these products will advertise that they are "all natural." Remember what we warned you about. "Natural" is not synonymous with harmless. Make sure that you are reading labels carefully and doing your research so that you know what you are putting into your body. Furthermore, to ensure that you know what you are getting, you should only buy from a company or brand that you trust; there have been a couple of "natural" products that were including ingredients that they hadn't listed on their label. Some had even laced their product with sildenafil (Viagra®), which is extremely dangerous to mix with some common blood pressure medications. A November 2007 Associated Press story on the topic reported that an Oregon research lab found that approximately 90 percent of the samples they had analyzed contained undisclosed patented pharmaceuticals.[21] Ever since the "snake oil" vendors of the 1800s, there have been people lined up to take your money for healthcare wonder cures. Beware of any product that claims it can "cure," has a "proprietary" blend, or can't offer any studies to back up their claims. Having said that, there are a lot of incredibly helpful herbs out there and the science to support them—you just need to learn how to educate yourself.

NUTRITION

Zinc is a mineral that is very important to men's health. Zinc is needed for the pituitary to release LH, which stimulates the testes to produce testosterone.[22] Zinc is involved in the suppression of aromatase, so it plays a huge role in protecting the prostate as well as maintaining healthy testosterone levels and sperm production. It is also needed by the enzyme that converts androstenedione (a precursor) into testosterone. Of course, these are just a few of the many roles that zinc plays in the body, and it is an important nutrient for everyone, but it's particularly important for men who are looking to enhance or optimize their hormonal health. You can find zinc in oysters, herring, wheat germ, pumpkin seeds, milk, crab, lobster, chicken, pork chops, turkey, lean ground beef, liver, and eggs. As you can see, if you are a vegetarian, you will likely need to make it a point to ensure you are getting enough zinc in your diet. A reasonable daily dosage would be 15 mg for long-term use. When you supplement zinc, there are a couple of important things to remember. Coffee will decrease the absorption of zinc by approximately 50 percent, so your dosage should be taken several hours away from your morning cup of joe, and you will need to supplement a small amount of copper to maintain the proper zinc-to-copper balance (which should be approximately 10:1). Zinc is a good example of a nutrient that teaches us the lesson that more is not always better. While small doses of zinc have been shown to enhance the immune system, larger doses (75 mg/day) may suppress long-term immunity.

Arginine is an amino acid that is nonessential, meaning that we don't have to get it from food—we can synthesize it in our bodies. Low arginine is associated with low sperm count, but more importantly, arginine boosts nitric oxide production and thus plays a role in cardiovascular health and healthy erections. Arginine is found in beans, brewer's yeast, chocolate, dairy, eggs, fish, legumes, meat, nuts, oatmeal, popcorn, raisins, seafood, sesame seeds, soy, sunflower seeds, whey, and whole grains. During times of stress, we don't produce as much arginine, so getting it from food becomes even more important. A typical supplemental dosage of arginine is 2 to 3 grams per day, though most people do not need to supplement it. One warning, though: if you have a history of herpes or cold sores, high levels of arginine may increase the likelihood of a breakout.

One of the factors in low testosterone is the suppression of its production by high cortisol levels. There is some evidence to support that the use of phosphatidylserine, a phospholipid found in your cell membranes, may help to blunt the elevated cortisol levels that occur when your body is subjected to an acute stressor such as a workout. What? Exercise is going to cause my testosterone levels to be suppressed? Overall, the testosterone producing aspects of exercise still far outweigh any suppression, not to mention the many other benefits of exercise. Studies have shown that cortisol levels are increased following a workout, and elevated cortisol has been linked to suppression of testosterone. A 600 mg/day dose of phosphatidylserine will blunt the increase in cortisol production,[23] but should only be done immediately following exercise as you do not want to suppress your cortisol production overall.

Carnitine is an amino acid that we can manufacture from the amino acids lysine and methionine, and it plays a large role in cardiovascular health, as well as a part in proper glucose utilization.[24] A recent study showed that carnitine was comparable with testosterone administration in the treatment of sexual dysfunction, fatigue, and depressed mood in aging men. Compared with placebo, carnitine proved to increase erection quality and ejaculation velocity as well as improve mood and energy; however, it was not shown to actually increase testosterone levels in serum.[25] The exact mechanism for all of this hasn't been detailed yet, but we do know that carnitine increases sperm motility when added to semen[26] and, therefore, is a recommended supplement for men who are suffering from infertility problems. Dosages for the purposes of increasing energy should be approximately 2 g/day.

We hope that after reading the last chapter you will be getting your vitamin D levels checked, and, if so, you will learn that you are likely low in this very important nutrient. Vitamin D is necessary for the proper functioning of the thyroid and pituitary glands (which, by proxy, makes it important for proper testosterone production). Vitamin D is also important for a number of other functions in the body including insulin sensitivity and protection from several forms of cancer. Food sources of vitamin D are cold-water fish, cod-liver oil, liver, and egg yolks. Many of our foods such as dairy and cereals are fortified with vitamin D, meaning that they have added it to that food, since the nutrient wasn't naturally occurring there. We make most of our vitamin D in our skin from sunlight, but depending on where you live, what time of the year it is, the color of your skin, and your use of sunscreen, you may not be getting nearly as much as you need. There is a minor controversy over the dosing of vitamin D. We recommend a daily supplement of 2,000 IU (international units) as a safe dose, and we frequently use much more than that with some patients. Of course, keeping your doctor in the loop is important: they can measure your 25-OH vitamin D3 levels and calcium while you are supplementing to make sure you are getting a healthy dose for your body.

Recent research has shown that men with high levels of soy intake had lower levels of estradiol, which is protective to the prostate. This is probably due to the inhibition of the aromatase enzyme by soy.[27] The essential fatty acids EPA and DHA (found in fish and cod-liver oil) decreased the levels of SHBG in men between the ages of 43 to 88.[28] Lower levels of SHBG will likely boost testosterone levels by making more of the testosterone bioavailable to the tissues. In addition to the vitamin D testing, we hope you have a chance to test your iodine levels. Iodine is a very important nutrient for proper thyroid function; however, iodine is also important to many tissues in your body including breast, prostate, and testicles. Iodine has been added to salt, which turns out to be the primary source of it for most Americans, but that isn't likely to be providing nearly as much as you need. Other sources of iodine include seaweed (especially kelp) and seafood. A common dosage ranges from 200 mcg to 12.5 mg (12,500 mcg). Many holistic healthcare providers recommend approximately 12.5 mg of iodine/iodide a day. This dosage is based on the average iodine intake in Japan of 13.8 mg. (In Japan, they have much lower incidence of thyroid and breast disease.) However, if you have thyroid disease or iodine sensitivity, extra caution should be used.

Selenium is a trace mineral that plays a role with the antioxidant glutathione peroxidase. It helps to protect against toxic pollutants including the elimination of arsenic and protection against the effects of cadmium and mercury.[29] Selenium appears to accumulate in the prostate and incite apoptosis (cell death) of the prostate cells, causing a cancer-protective effect.[30] Selenium also plays a large role in thyroid health, and, in fact, the thyroid is the place in the body where we see selenium the most concentrated. The mineral is required for the conversion of T4 (the inactive, circulating form of thyroid hormone) to T3, the bio-available form of thyroid hormone.[31] This conversion is imperative to thyroid and all endocrine health. Dosages of approximately 400 mcg/day are appropriate.

Chromium is another trace mineral that is very important in maintaining proper insulin sensitivity, and, it may help to shift body composition from fat to more lean body mass. This nutrient is particularly important to those of you who feel as though metabolic syndrome is part of your picture: you have hypoglycemic episodes, have a tendency to store weight around your midsection, or maybe have been told that your blood sugar levels are a little high. Chromium is found in brewer's yeast, blackstrap molasses, black pepper, meat, whole wheat breads and cereals, broccoli, cheese, nut legumes, beets, and mushrooms. Dosages of 200 to 400 micrograms a day are recommended.

In addition to the nutritional compounds that support and enhance optimal testosterone production, there are a number of vitamins, minerals, and amino acid supplements that can help to stimulate growth hormone production. Vitamin A is believed to affect IGF-3, which is needed to produce growth hormone. Recommended dosage is approximately 3,000 to 6,000 IU/day of vitamin A. Gamma Aminobutyric Acid (GABA) is another nonessential amino acid and an abundant neurotransmitter that has been found to stimulate growth hormone, particularly when taken after exercise. A dose of 200 to 600 mg/day is reasonable; however, it can cause some sleepiness, so beware if taking it in the morning or the middle of a busy day. Glutamine, an amino acid that is abundant in muscle and cells in your gastrointestinal tract, is believed to exert a direct stimulation of growth hormone. Tryptophan is an essential amino acid that we get from bananas, beans, brewer's yeast, dairy products, dates, eggs, fish, legumes, meat, nuts, seafood, soy, and many whole grains. Tryptophan is not currently available as a supplement; however, 5 hydroxytryptophan (5-HTP), a close relative, is available and can exert the many effects of tryptophan including boosting the release of growth hormone.

Indole-3-carbinol (I3C) and diindolylmethane (DIM) are compounds that are found in cruciferous vegetables such as broccoli, brussel sprouts, cabbage, and kale. These phytonutrients are protective against estrogen-mediated conditions such as benign prostatic hypertrophy (BPH) and prostate cancer[32] and can help your body metabolize estrogens more quickly. ICD and DIM may also play a role in cellular communication and prevent existing cancer from metastasizing to other tissues.[33] So eat your vegetables, and regardless of your opinion of George Bush, Sr. don't follow in his footsteps in avoiding broccoli, as it's a very nutritious vegetable and may prevent you from developing cancer!

LIFESTYLE

Exercise, exercise, exercise. Ok, so you know that exercise is good for you, but what kind of exercise, when, and for how long? Of course, it depends on what you are trying to do. If you want to win the Tour de France, you should focus on endurance exercises that will help your body make it over those mountains in the Alps. Actually, testosterone levels can decline as a result of strenuous, endurance-style exercise. Aerobic and anaerobic exercise increases your testosterone levels initially, but if the workout exceeds about two hours, the stress on your body causes testosterone levels to fall.[34] If you want to boost your testosterone, you should go for shorter, more intense workouts.[35] Specifically, resistance exercise has been shown to increase testosterone levels.[36] Weight training has been reported to improve testosterone levels, and general consensus seems to be that you should be getting at least three hours a week of moderately intensive exercise, but not overdoing it. That boils down to 30 minutes a day of an intense workout, and you can still rest on Sunday and watch football.

Speaking of football watching on Sunday, many of you are likely putting down a few beers during those games. You should really be limiting your intake to one or two drinks at a time to avoid causing a decrease in testosterone levels. Shedding a few pounds will likely boost your testosterone levels as well. We discussed the relationship between abdominal weight and testosterone levels earlier in this book, and they certainly have a relationship where they each affect each other. Increasing your testosterone levels will likely cause you to shed a few pounds and increase lean body mass and conversely, losing a few inches can increase your testosterone levels.

As you can see, there are a number of dietary supplements, nutritional components, and lifestyle changes you can add to your life to enhance your production of testosterone and growth hormone, slow your manufacturing of estrogen, and help prevent various forms of cancer. In approximately 400 BC, the father of Western medicine, Hippocrates, stated, "May your food be your medicine and your medicine be your food." Think about it. Your body can only be as good as the fuel you put in it. If you were to skimp a little at the gas pump and put a low-octane fuel in your car, you'd likely notice the difference. Many of us are routinely providing our bodies with "fuel" that would be analogous to an "octane" level far below what we should be using. Yet we don't seem to take action when we notice "knocking and pinging" in our bodies. If you are suffering from many of the symptoms detailed in this book, then we recommend you take the necessary steps to restore your hormones to optimal levels and prevent further decline. This will likely be a combination of actions including cleaning up your diet, increasing your exercise, and possibly optimizing your testosterone levels through bioidentical testosterone supplementation. If you are one of the lucky men reading this that hasn't yet seen or felt the effects of declining hormone levels, then take action now! There are so many things that you can do to **prevent** many of these problems from occurring prematurely. Yes, it's true, as we've told you, your testosterone levels will drop as you age regardless of what you do, but your goal should be to produce your own hormones as long for as you can!

NOTES

1. Ang, H. and K. Lee, "Effect of Eurycoma longifolia Jack on orientation activities in middle-aged male rats," *Fundam Clin Pharmacol* (2004) 16;479–83. Ang, H. and H. Cheang, "Effects of Eurycoma longifolia jack (Tongkat ali) on the initiation of sexual performance of inexperienced castrated male rats," *Exp Amin* (2000) 49:35–38.

2. Gauthaman, K. and A.P. Ganesan, "The hormonal effects of Tribulus terrestris and its role in the management of male erectile dysfunction—an evaluation using primates, rabbit and rat," *Phytomedicine* (2008) Jan;15(1–2):44–54. Gauthaman, K., A.P. Ganesan, R.N.V. Prasad, "Sexual effects of puncturevine (Tribulus terrestris) extract (Protodioscin): An evaluation using a rat model," *The Journal of Alternative and Complementary Medicine* (2003) April 1;9(2):257–265.

3. Cirigliano, M.D. and P.O. Szapary, "Horny goat weed for erectile dysfunction," *Alt Med Alert* (2001) 4:19–22.

4. Schottner, M., D. Gansser, G. Spiteller, "Lignans from the roots of Urtica dioica and their metabolites bind on human sex hormone binding globulin (SHBG)," *Plana Med* (1997) Dec;63(6):529–32.

5. Kellis, J.T. Jr and L.E. Vickery, "Inhibition of human estrogen synthetase (aromatase) by flavones," *Science* (1984) Wep 7;225(4666):1032–4.

6. Wang, C., et al, "Lignans and flavonoids inhibit aromatase enzyme in human preadipocytes," *J Steroid Biochem Mol Biol* (1994) 50:205–12.

7. Shimoi, K., et al, "Intestinal absorption of luteolin 7-O-beta-glucoside in rats and humans," FEBS Lett (1998) 438:220–24.

8. Di Silverio, F., S. Monti, A. Sciarra, P.A. Varasano, C. Martini, S. Lanzara, G. D'Eramo, S. Di Nicola, V. Toscoano, "Effects of long-term treatment with Serenoa repens (Permixon®) on the concentrations and regional distribution of androgens and epidermal growth factor in benign prostatic hyperplasia."

9. Carraro, J.C., J.P. Raynoud, G. Koch, et al, "Comparison of phytotherapy (Permixon®) with finasteride in the treatment of benign prostate hyperplasia: A randomized international study of 1,098 patients," *Prostate* (1996) 29:231–40.

10. Li, G., U. Ammermann, C.F. Quiros, "Gluconsinolate contents in Maca (Lepidiumperuvianum Chacon) seeds, sprouts, mature plants, and several derived commercial products," *Economic Botany* (2001) 55:255–62.

11. Law, M, "Plant sterol and stanol margarines and health," *BMJ* (2000) 320:861–4.

12. Cabeza, M., E. Bratoeff, I. Heuze, et al, "Effect of beta-sitosterol as inhibitor of 5 alpha-reductase in hamster prostate," *Proc West Pharmacol Soc* (2003) 46:153–5.

13. Hiipakka, R.A., "Structure-activity relationships for inhibition of human 5 alpha-reductases by polyphenols," *Biochem Pharmacol* (2002) Mar 15;63(6):1165–76.

14. Lee, J., "Prostate disease and hormones," The John R. Lee, MD Medical Letter, Feb. 2002.

15. Hetts, S, "To die or not to die: an overview of apoptosis and its role in disease," JAMA (1998) 279:300–07.

16. Yablonsky, F., V. Nicolas, J.P. Riffaud, F. Bellamy, "Antiproliferative effect of Pygeum africanum extract on rat prostatic fibroblasts," *J Urol* (1997) 157:2881–7.

17. Duke, James A., *CRC Handbook of Medicinal Herbs*, (CRC Press, Inc., 1985).

18. Waynberg, J., "Male sexual asthenia—interest in a traditional plan-derived medication," *Ethnopharmacology* (1995) Mar.

19. Choi, Y.D., Z.C. Xin, H.K. Choi, "Effect of Korean red ginseng on the rabbit corpus cavernosal smooth muscle," *Int J Impot Res* (1998) 10:37–43.

Kim, H.J., D.S. Woo, G. Lee, J.J. Kim, "The relaxation effects of ginseng saponin in rabbit corporal smooth muscle: is it a nitric oxide donor?" *Br J Urol* (1998) 82:744–748.

20. Choi, H.K., D.H. Seong, K.H. Rha, "Clinical efficacy of Korean red ginseng for erectile dysfunction," *Int J Impot Res* (1995) 7:181–186.

21. *Report: Popping Herbal Sex Pills Linked to Increased Risk of Stroke, Headaches, Vision Problems*, Associated Press, November 13, 2007 (http://www.foxnews.com/story/0,2933,310936,00.html).

22. Hunt, C.D., P.E. Johnson, J.L. Hebel, L.K. Mullen, "Effects of dietary zinc depletion on seminal volume and zinc loss, serum testosterone concentrations, and sperm morphology in young men," *Am J Clin Nutr* (1992) 56:148–57.

23. Starks, M.A., S.L. Starks, M. Kingsley, M. Purpura, R. Jager, "The effects of phosphatidylserine on endocrine response to moderate intensity exercise," *Journal of the International Society of Sports Nutrition* (2008) 5:11.

24. Mingrone, G., "Carnitine in type 2 diabetes," *Ann NY Acad Sci* (2004) 1033:99–107.

25. Cavallini, G., S. Caracciolo, G. Vitali, F. Modenini, G. Biagiotti, "Carnitine versus androgen administration in the treatment of sexual dysfunction, depressed mood, and fatigue associated with male aging," *Urology* (2004) Apr;63(4):641–6.

26. Tanphaichitr, N., "In vitro stimulation of human sperm motility by acetylcarnitine," *Int J Fertil* (1977) 22:85–91.

27. Nagata, C., S. Inaba, N. Kawakami, T. Kakizoe, H. Shimizu, "Inverse association of soy product intake with serum androgen and estrogen concentrations in Japanese men," *Nutr Cancer* (2000) 36(1):14–8.

28. Nagata, C., N. Takatsuka, N. Kawakami, H. Shimizu, "Relationships between types of fat consumed and serum estrogen and androgen concentrations in Japanese men," *Nutr Cancer* (2000) 38(2):163–67.

29. Klatz, Goldman, *The Official Anti-Aging Revolution.*

30. Taylor, P.R., H.L. Parnes, S.M. Lippman, "Science peels the onion of selenium effects on prostate carcinogenesis," *J Natl Cancer Inst* (2004) 96:645–7.

31. Neve, J., "New approaches to assess selenium status and requirement," *Nutr Rev* (2000) 58:363–9.

32. Michnovicz, J.J. and H.L. Bradlow, "Induction of esradiol metabolism by dietary indole-3-carbinol in humans," *J Natl Cancer Inst* (1992) Aug 5;84(15):1210–2.

33. Hsu, E.L., N. Chen, A. Westbrook, F. Wang, R. Zhang, R.T. Taylor, O. Hankinson, "CXCR4 and CXCL12 down-regulation: a novel mechanism for the chemoprotection of 3,3'-diindolylmethane for breast and ovarian cancers," *Cancer Lett* (2008) Jun 28;265(1):113–23.

34. Hackney, A.C., "Endurance exercise training and reproductive endocrine dysfunction in men: alterations in the hypothalamic-pituitary-testicular axis." Hackney, A.C., E. Szczepanowska, A.M. Viru, "Basal testicular testosterone production in endurance-trained men is suppressed," *Eur J Appl Physiol* (2003) Apr 89(2):198–201.

35. Eliakim, A. and D. Nemet, "Exercise and the male reproductive system," *Harefuah* (2006) Sep 145(9):677–81,702,701.

36. Schumm, S.R., N.T. Triplett, J.M. McBride, C.L. Dumke, "Hormonal response to carbohydrate supplementation at rest and after resistance exercise," *Int J Sport Nutr Exerc Metab* (2008) Jun 18(3):260–80.

CHAPTER 10

Protective Steps

So, what can you do to protect yourself from the effects of declining testosterone levels? Depending on your age, you may not be suffering from the heart disease, diabetes, depression, fatigue, and/or erectile dysfunction associated with low testosterone levels... **yet**. Or maybe you

> "An ounce of prevention is worth a pound of cure."—Benjamin Franklin

are experiencing many of these problems, but want to keep your sons or nephews or younger brothers from having to go through it. It's never too late or too early to start living a healthier lifestyle. Many of the same things that will increase your testosterone levels (if they are below where they should be) are also helpful to keep them from falling in the first place! In a football game, you will find that you don't need a "Hail Mary" in the final seconds if you have executed your offensive and defensive plays well throughout the game. Many of the same steps that will protect your levels from unnecessarily falling in the first place may help to repair and restore those who find themselves in the middle of the game already.

One of the first things you can do is to keep your body fat levels low, but not too low. Total body fat percentage should ideally be at or below 20 percent, but not below 5 percent. There is a lot of information available out there regarding the dangers of low body fat percentage for women, but not as many studies have been done for men. There have been a couple of studies done with wrestlers, because this is one population that tends to cut their weight dramatically and drop their body fat. One study showed that low testosterone levels were correlated with low body fat as well as rapid weight loss.[1] You probably know how much you weigh, but you may be wondering how you measure body fat? The "gold standard" is a

Body Fat Percentage		
Level	Men	Women
Optimal	6-14%	16-23%
Acceptable	15-25%	24-32%
Obese	Over 25%	Over 32%

process called hydrodensitometry, which is really just a fancy word for underwater weighing. This is done by weighing the patient, and then immersing them totally in water and weighing them again. Bones and muscle are more dense than fat, so a person with more body fat will weigh comparatively less in the pool than a person with more muscle and bone. This method is employed in many spas and health clubs, but is not simple for the average guy to do at home. Another commonly employed method is the measurement of subcutaneous fat (that means fat under your skin) with skinfold calipers. The calipers measure the thickness of the fat at various places on the body and an equation is used to estimate overall total body fat. This method is also used in many gyms, but lends itself to a small degree of subjectivity, as the results can vary depending on the person measuring. Still another way of assessing body fat is through a process called bioelectrical impedance analysis (BIA).

BIA runs a small electrical current through the body from two conductors and measures the resistance between the two. Adipose tissue is a poor conductor of electrical current, whereas muscle is full of electrolytes and conducts electricity well. This used to require special equipment, but there are now many affordable scales on the market that use two conductor pads that attach to each foot to assess body fat percentage. It can now be done in your own home! For those of you who aren't starting this "getting healthy" process with a clean slate and want to know what your current body fat percentage means, the table above can let you know where you fall currently and help you set some goals.

Don't let the following recommendations cause you to scratch your head. We know that we just told you to try to get (and keep) your body fat percentage down, but it's also important to make sure that you are eating sufficient protein and fat. Research has shown that a low-fat diet will cause testosterone production to decline.[2] Yep, first we told you that we wanted you to lower your body fat, and now we're telling you to eat fat. But, you are what you eat, right? Well, kind of. Not all fats are created equal. We know, everywhere you go there are advertisements for low-fat foods. You've been force-fed the idea that fats were bad for a long time. By all means, you should be avoiding hydrogenated fats and partially hydrogenated fats. Hydrogenation is a process where fats are modified to give them a longer shelf life. Sounds like a good idea, except that the process creates a version of fats called trans fats that your body can't process, so not only are we missing out on the valuable nutritional benefits of fat, the fats we are eating are having an additional negative impact on our health because these synthetic compounds **cause** a number of problems in your body.

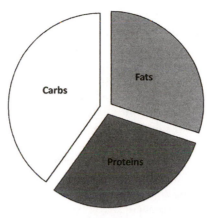

Figure 10.1 Your diet should include approximately 30% fat, 30% protein and 40% carbohydrates.

You are likely familiar with some of these dangers, as trans fats have been increasingly named in the media and are even being banned in some cities. Unfortunately, if you're a fan of fried foods as so many of us are, this is bad news. Most fried foods, especially at restaurants, are fried in partially hydrogenated vegetable oil. Read your labels, and you will find partially hydrogenated vegetable oils in just about all prepackaged foods. These fats are toxic and interfere with the roles that "good fats" play in your body. The fats we want you to consume are things like olive oil, fish oil, sunflower oil, and coconut oil. There are many different kinds of fats: omega-3s, omega-6s, omega-9s, and saturated fats. You may be familiar with some of these. As a general guideline, your diet should consist of approximately 30 percent fat, 30 percent protein, and 40 percent carbohydrates. Take a look at your diet. Even if you're careful with carbohydrates (in light of the reputation that they have developed), it's likely that they account for more than 40 percent of your intake. And of the 30 percent of your diet that's made from fats, most of it (about 60 percent) should be from monounsaturated fats such as olive oil; 30 percent from saturated fats such as coconut oil, butter, raw dairy, and animal fats; and 10 percent from polyunsaturated fats such as fish oil, flax seed oil, sunflower oil, or sesame oil.

These guidelines are just that, to guide you. But sticking relatively close to this should ensure that you won't be adversely affecting your testosterone levels. Protein is another important dietary factor when it comes to hormone levels. Unless you have kidney or heart problems or have been told by a doctor to watch your intake of protein for another reason, we would recommend that you aim for approximately 0.7 grams of protein for every 2 pounds you weigh. So if you weigh 200 pounds, then you would divide 200 by 2 and multiply by 0.7. Thus, 200/2 = 100 and 100 × 0.7 = **70 grams per day**. Protein in your diet will increase muscle mass, help your body control its cortisol levels, and keep your testosterone levels from dropping. Just a warning though, in high-protein diets such as Atkins, there is a reduction in testosterone levels.[3] So while you want to consume a healthy amount of protein, your diet should always consist of a greater percentage of carbohydrates than protein, as long as those carbohydrates aren't all in the form of pure sugar and processed foods. And, as always, you need to be careful and pay attention to the sources of your protein. Because most of the animals we eat for protein are near the top of the food chain, they are often from places where pesticides and chemicals can be concentrated. Local, organic meats and fish are your best bet. As a general rule, the closer you can get to actually meeting the animal you are going to eat, the better.

With all of these changes to your diet, you are likely to lose weight, if you have it to lose. There's nothing wrong with that. There are many connections between low testosterone levels and high body weight. While you should optimize your weight, you shouldn't lose it too quickly. Weight loss should be limited to one to two pounds a week. If you cut your caloric intake by more than 15 percent, your body will act as though it's starving and testosterone levels will decline.[4] When your body perceives that it's starving, it goes into storage mode and will shut down the production of testosterone and sperm because they require energy to produce, and testosterone doesn't play a role in feeding the body. Remember when we talked about your body's ability to establish a hierarchy of what is important for survival? When the threat is something scary chasing you, your body shifts focus to the fight or flight response and gives blood and energy to the large muscles that will help you run, and to the heart and lungs to keep oxygen flowing. If the threat is starvation, the body will shift focus to the storage of energy in the form of fat and glycogen production. Glycogen is the storage form of glucose. Unfortunately, neither of the previous two situations requires much help from the testicles, so they receive a decrease in blood and stimulation which results in decreased testosterone levels. Dramatic caloric restriction can cause this starving reaction as well as "fasting" periods, or lengths of time without food. For this reason, you should eat five to six small meals throughout the day, spaced evenly apart, and make sure that you start with breakfast; this will provide your body with the nutrients it needs, and prevent it from perceiving that you are starving.

Exercise, especially weight-bearing exercise, can help to keep your testosterone levels in optimal range. Heavy resistance training has been shown to increase testosterone levels in both young (23 to 35 years old) and less young (58 to 65 years old) men.[5] Multijoint exercises such as the squat, bench press, seated row, and lat pull-down affect testosterone levels more than smaller muscle group exercises. When lifting, you should push yourself: the greatest increase in testosterone levels will come from 70 percent to 85 percent of your one rep max, which should allow you about five repetitions and no more. Furthermore, three sets at this level will stimulate the most testosterone production. Of course, you should always make sure you are giving your muscles a full day to recover. Rest between heavy workouts is very important.[6] You don't need an exclusive gym membership or own an expensive weight machine to do resistance exercises. There are a number of things you can do with a simple set of weights or resistance bands set up in your garage, spare room, or office.

While exercise and food are important, many people have a hard time implementing those changes into their schedules and lives for a number of reasons. We know it is hard work to change your lifestyle. So, here's some advice that should be easy to follow: why don't you sleep in a bit, and reward your hard work with some "quality time" with your partner? Yes, by "quality time," we're referring to sex. First, you should make sure you are getting enough sleep. Seven to eight hours a night is ideal. Poor sleep or lack of sleep can cause your testosterone levels to fall significantly.[7] Sleep allows your whole body, including your hormone producing glands, the necessary time to experience "restoration." After all, the first four letters in restoration are R-E-S-T. You need rest as much as you need activity to help keep your body working optimally. Growth hormone is released while you are sleeping, and lack of sleep will cause cortisol levels to rise, so there are a number of good reasons why you should sleep in! And if you do make it out of bed with a few extra minutes in the morning, you should try to squeeze in some morning sex. Did you know that you can actually boost your testosterone levels by having sex, and even from simply getting an erection?[8] So, making time for a "quickie" in the morning can give you a big boost for the entire day!

You are probably familiar with the effects that alcohol can have on erections, as many of you have likely found yourself a little less prepared than you thought you were (or wanted to be) for a sexual encounter after having a few drinks. In addition to affecting your erections, alcohol can suppress your production of testosterone so you should limit yourself to three alcoholic drinks per day.[9] And just to clarify, for those of you who may be inclined to consider a 28 oz stein as one drink, a drink is defined as 1.5 oz of liquor (at approximately 40 percent alcohol or 80 proof), 5 oz of wine (11 percent alcohol), or 12 oz of beer (4 percent alcohol).[10] If your drink of choice has a high alcohol content, such as many microbrews or fortified wines, then the beverage count needs to be adjusted accordingly.

When we were covering the many theories and actions of aging, we discussed the role of antioxidants briefly. Antioxidants are molecules that help to slow down or stop the oxidation process, which basically helps you and your cells become more "rust-proof." We used the example of rust earlier when we were explaining oxidation, since it's one that many of you have likely experienced. The oxidation process is a natural one, and serves many purposes in the body including an important role in the innate immune reaction; however, there is a dark side to these substances, and they can wreak havoc on our bodies.[11] Many of our immune cells will release free radicals as defense against foreign substances. These free radicals or pro-oxidants are powerful and work to destroy the pathogen in question. This is an effective and very important part of our immune reaction, but there can be repercussions because the free radicals can work to destroy other tissues as well. Antioxidants are compounds that can stop the cascade of free radicals that are likely responsible for several diseases and many of the effects of aging.[12] Most antioxidants come from fruits and vegetables, and you will get more antioxidant properties the less the plant is cooked. Not all antioxidants are found in the diet; however, some compounds are produced in our bodies including glutathione and coenzyme Q10. Some antioxidants are water soluble, while others mix better in lipids or fats. A mixture of the two is important so that you are protecting all parts of your cells. A few of the "big name" antioxidants include vitamin C, vitamin A, vitamin E, alpha lipoic acid, and flavonoids such as lycopene or resveratrol. Making sure that you have a healthy dose of antioxidants in your diet will protect all of your tissues (including your pituitary gland and your testicles) from free-radical damage. Ideally, it is always best to eat plenty of fresh vegetables and fruits because getting these nutrients from food sources is the best place to start.

Some of the things that you can do to prevent your testosterone levels from dropping faster than they would otherwise aren't things to do at all, but are rather things not to do. There are a lot of things that you should avoid due to their effects on your body, and your hormone levels in particular. Let's start with pesticides. You've likely wondered if this whole craze about organic foods is worth all the fuss. Is it really worth $5 a pound for **organic** strawberries or would you be ok just picking up the cheapest thing you can find? If you were given an opportunity to fill up your car for 99 cents a gallon, you would probably question the deal and wonder about the quality of the product and whether it might harm your engine. Why treat your body any differently? With few exceptions in this world, you mostly get what you pay for. It's rare to see a good deal on something of quality on an ongoing basis; it is just not economically sustainable. Yet, how many 99 cent food deals are there at fast food restaurants? Many people who question the quality of the products that they put into their cars or their homes think nothing of filling themselves up with "99 cent fuel." Your health should be the last place you are trying to "get a deal"!

We recommend that you be very careful about the chemicals you are putting in your body, and where your food comes from. Pesticides are created to kill pests, and pests are basically anything that interferes with the crops, availability to humans. This can include molds, bacteria, insects, worms, weeds, and even animals that may eat or otherwise interfere with the plants. So we spray our **food** with these chemicals that kill other living organisms. Did you know that scientists frequently use the DNA of fruit flies to study aspects of human genetics because we share such a large number of genes? In fact, about 75 percent of the genes that we know code for diseases in humans are also found in the fruit fly.[13] What does this have to do with anything? The point is that we have more in common with other organisms, including those that are as different from us as a fly, than we ever thought. No wonder those chemicals that are designed to kill insects and bacteria have an adverse affect on our cells as well. So what kinds of effects do these pesticides have? Well, the effects are as varied as the substances used. For our purposes, we're particularly interested in the chemicals that disrupt endocrine pathways and affect testosterone levels, although you could end up with leukemia, Parkinson's disease, or worse. Organophosphates, a large category of pesticides that are related to the nerve gas Sarin, have many toxic effects including disturbing testosterone synthesis.[14] Even if you wash your fruits and vegetables, if there are pesticides in the soil, then it will turn up in them both. Thanks to modern technology and modern transportation, we eat food that literally comes from all over the world. It's hard to know what standards are applied in other countries; they may be using extremely toxic compounds. We recommend that you try to buy fruits and vegetables from local sources, and ask questions about what chemicals they have used on or near the plants. And, of course, always wash your fruits and vegetables.

Another classification of chemicals called polychlorinated biphenyls (PCBs) have been used as plasticizers and coolants, and used in sealants, adhesives, waterproofing compounds, and pesticides. These compounds have found their way into our soil and water, and are especially concentrated in animals higher on the food chain. We are likely exposed to many of these compounds daily, and they have also been shown to adversely affect testosterone levels in men.[15] How do you avoid PCBs? Well, you should probably not eat fish from lakes or water sources that are near factories. The Great Lakes, for example, have been implicated as having high PCB levels. Avoiding solvents, especially older compounds, and old electrical transformers or old industrial sites is also a good idea.

Speaking of all of these chemicals that we can inadvertently be exposed to, we can't forget to mention one of the most common exposures to toxic chemicals: cigarettes. Really, you've seen the commercials, you've read the headlines, and you know it's not good for you. So why do so many people still smoke? We wish we knew. Seriously, the list of chemicals in cigarettes is staggering. We could go through them one by one and detail the adverse affects of most of them, but we'd need another couple of hundred pages. In fact, many of the chemicals you find in cigarettes come from the tobacco plant being sprayed with pesticides before being dried and rolled into that neat little wrapper. So, the chemicals we have been talking about avoiding end up being sucked into the fragile lung tissue. Though we can't talk about them all, we do want to highlight one of the nearly 4,000 chemicals and substances that can be isolated from tobacco. Cadmium is a metal that is found naturally in the earth, but in small amounts. Cigarette smoke is the primary place where people are exposed to cadmium, and its effects are certainly negative. Cadmium has been shown to—you guessed it—lower testosterone levels in rat studies.[16] But that's not all. Cadmium has also been implicated in prostate cancer,[17] lung cancer, and high blood pressure.[18]

Another big area of chemical exposure is in cosmetics and personal care products. We know, you probably don't wear makeup, but we're talking broadly of the cosmetic industry. This includes face lotions, shaving creams and gels, shampoos, and even personal lubricants. Are you with us now? You probably use some of these products, and you should check your labels carefully and avoid those products that contain parabens. Parabens are a group of chemicals that are used as preservatives in products such as those listed. There is still a mild controversy regarding the safety of these compounds, and so for now they are still ubiquitous. Studies on whether or not parabens have anti-androgen consequences have been done, and there was a correlation shown; however, these studies were preliminary and further research is warranted.[19]

Alright, we think you get the picture about some of the many possible places you can be exposed to chemicals and at least some of the things that they can do to your body. So don't be too macho to wear protective gear when it's necessary.

> To get rich never risk your health. For it is the truth that health is the wealth of wealth.
> —Richard Baker

Gloves can protect your skin from absorbing a number of chemicals, masks can prevent inhalation of dust particles that are laden with harmful chemicals, and proper clothing will keep any splashing or spilling of substances from touching your skin. You don't have to wear a hazmat suit to work every day (unless you literally work with hazardous materials), but you should be careful. And while you will inadvertently be exposed to a number of things, you can help to lessen the burden on your body by making sure that you are eliminating toxins. How can you do that? Two words: poop more. How many times a day do you visit that toilet? Ideally, you should be having two to three bowel movements every day. If this isn't the case, you should take a look at your fiber intake. A good goal is to try to eat thirty to forty grams of fiber a day. There are two types of fiber, soluble and insoluble. Soluble fiber will bind to toxins, as well as cholesterol and excess hormones, and help to remove them from your system. Insoluble fiber provides bulk to help attract water and move things through your colon. You can think of insoluble fiber as a big broom that "cleans" you out. Most sources of fiber have both components present; the insoluble fiber is usually the skin, hull, or rind of the fruit or grain; a good example of soluble fiber would be the pectin inside the apple. Of course you will need to make sure that you are drinking plenty of water with the fiber you eat, as you don't want to create a "beaver dam" effect in your colon.

One more thing that you can do to help keep your testicles pumping out that testosterone: reduce your stress level. We've said it several times, because we know that this is a big factor in the decline of so many people's health. We are literally running ourselves into the ground. That chronic stress scenario that we've been talking about is responsible for so many health problems; digestive disorders, body aches and pains, anxiety and depression, endocrine disruptions, and memory problems can all be caused by or exacerbated by stress. So if you want to prevent your testosterone levels from dropping, then chill out. Learn to deal with your stress, slow down, exercise, take a vacation, have sex, take a nap, and ultimately prioritize what matters: your health.

NOTES

1. Strauss, R.H., R.R. Lanese, W.B. Marlarkey, "Weight loss in amateur wrestlers and its effect on serum testosterone levels," *JAMA* (1985) Dec 20;254(23):3337–8.

2. Wang, C., D.H. Catlin, B. Starcevic, D. Heber, C. Ambler, N. Berman, G. Lucas, A. Leung, K. Schramm, P.W. Lee, L. Hull, R.S. Swerdloff, "Low-fat high-fiber diet decreased serum and urine androgens in men," *J Clin Endocrinol Metab* (2005) Jun; 90(6):3802.

Hamalainen, E., H. Aldercreutz, P. Puska, P. Pietinen, "Diet and serum sex hormones in healthy men," *J Steroid Biochem* (1984) Jan 20(1):459–64.

3. Anderson, K.E., W. Rosner, M.S. Khan, M.I. New, S.Y. Pang, P.S. Wissel, A. Kappas, "Diet-hormone interactions: protein/carbohydrate ration alters reciprocally the plasma levels of testosterone and cortisol and their respective binding globulins in man," *Life-Sci* (1987) May 4; 40(18):1761–8.

4. Klibanski, A., I.Z. Beitins, T. Badger, R. Little, J.W. McArthur, "Reproductive function during fasting in men," *J Clin Endocrinol Metab* (1981) Aug;53(2):258–63. Garrel, D.R. and K.S. Todd, "Pugeat MM. Calloway DH. Hormonal changes in normal men under marginally negative energy balance," *American Journal of Clinical Nutrition* (1984) Jun 39(6):930–6.

5. Kraemer, W.J., K. Hakkinen, R.U. Newoton, et al, "Effects of heavy-resistance training on hormonal response patterns in younger vs. older men," *J App Physiol* (1999) Sep 87(3):982–92.

6. Zinczenko, D. and T. Spiker, *The Abs Diet* (Rodale, Inc., 2004).

7. Luboshitzky, R., Z. Zabari, Z. Shen-Orr, P. Herer, P. Lavie, "Disruption of the nocturnal testosterone rhythm by sleep fragmentation in normal men," *J Clin Endocrinol Metab* (2001) Mar; 86(3):1134–9.

8. Sapolsky, R., "Vitamin T for Sex," WebMD, Oct. 16, 2000.

9. TaTaniguchi, N. and S.Kaneko, "Alcoholic effect on male sexual function," *Nippon Rinsho* (1997) Nov; 55(11):3040–4.

10. National Institute on Alcohol Abuse and Alcoholism, No. 16, PH 315, April 1992.

11. D.T. Sawyer, Superoxide Chemistry, Vol 17, McGraw-Hill Encyclopedia of Science & Technology, McGraw Hill Higher Education, 2002.

12. Bonnefoy, M., J. Drai J, T. Kostka, "Antioxidants to slow aging, facts and perspectives," *Presse Med* (2002) Jul 27;31(25):1174–84.

13. Reiter, L.T., L. Potocki, S. Chien, M. Gribskov, E. Bier, "A systematic analysis of human disease-associated gene sequences in drosophila melanogaster," *Genome Res* (2001) Jun; 11:1114–1125.

14. Contreras, H.R., V. Paredes, B. Urquieta, L. DelValle, E. Bustos-Obregon, "Testosterone production and spermatogenic damage induced by organophosphorate pesticides," *Biocell* (Mendoza), ago./dic. 2006; 30(3): 423–429.

15. Goncharov, A., "Association between serum polychlorinated biphenyls, pesticides and testosterone levels in a Native American Population," University of Albany.

16. Laskey, J.W., G.L. Rehnberg, S.C. Laws, J.F. Hein, "Reproductive effects of low acute doses of dacmium chloride in adult male rats," *Toxicol Appl Pharmacol* (1984) Apr;73(2):250–5.

17. Multigner, L., J.R. Ndong, A. Oliva, P. Blanchet, "Environmental pollutants and prostate cancer: epidemiological data," *Gynecol Obstet Fertil* (2008) Sep; 36(9):848–56.

18. Lee, J.S. and K.L. White, "A review of the health effects of cadmium," *American Journal of Industrial Medicine*, 1(3-4):307–317.

19. Chen, J., K.C. Ahn, N.A. Gee, S.J. Gee, B.D. Hammock, B.L. Lasley, "Antiandrogenic properties of parabens and other phenolic containing small molecules in personal care products," *Toxicol Appl Pharmacol* (2007) Jun 15;221(3):278–84.

Conclusion

We have made every effort to translate the science of the male body and hormonal influences into English. There are many proactive things you can do, but remember to keep your doctors in the loop. We hope that, by now, we have convinced you that hormones aren't just a factor in the lives of women. Both genders have all of the same hormones even though they are found in different amounts. The effect they have is just as important in the male body as it is in the female body. There are many roles that testosterone, estrogen, progesterone, cortisol, DHEA, and others play in your body from birth and development, through puberty, and into adulthood. Testosterone is a particularly important hormone when it comes to men's health as it is the primary androgen hormone that is responsible for male characteristics. Unfortunately, testosterone levels begin to decline after the age of 30, and for each decade men lose roughly 10 percent of their total testosterone levels. This problem is compounded by the fact that estrogen and sex hormone binding globulin levels rise with age, further reducing the free testosterone or the amount of the hormone that is available to bind to tissues. In addition, many diet and lifestyle choices make things even worse by driving testosterone levels down even further, increasing estrogen levels or altering body composition. Low or less-than-optimal testosterone levels can cause a number of problems in the body including fatigue, depression, metabolic syndrome, decrease in muscle tone, emotional lability, erectile dysfunction, and decreased mental capacity, just to name a few!

The modern medical community is well aware of the presence and purpose of testosterone and other hormones in men's bodies; yet, for the most part, it fails to recognize that the decline of these hormones is a real problem. Defining (and naming) the phenomenon of changing hormone levels in **women** was done years ago, yet there is some controversy regarding this similar process in men, and there is still no commonly used terminology. The bottom line is that we are living much longer than we ever did in years past, and this fact is revealing many changes that the human body undergoes through aging. We have extended our lives by almost 30 years over the course of the last four generations, yet by ignoring the change in hormone levels, we are extending the **quantity** of life, yet not necessarily the **quality**. What we need is a paradigm shift, a change in the way that we look at aging and health. This is your opportunity not only to shape the course and quality of your life, but to be a part of a greater movement of **proactive** health.

> "There is always some specific moment when we become aware that our youth is gone; but years after, we know it was much later."
> —Mignon McLaughlin

Andropause doesn't happen overnight, or even as quickly as menopause. It's a slow and sneaky decline of hormone levels that lures men into aging prematurely. Andropause is certainly not an event that waits until you are "old." Testosterone levels start to decline by age 30 and continue a steady drop of more than 1 percent each year after that. One percent may not sound like much, but just imagine how a pinhole in your gasoline tank would eventually drain your tank completely, one drop at a time. At the rate of 10 percent loss per decade, that leaves men in their seventies with just over half of the testosterone levels that they had when they were in their twenties. To some of you reading this, 70 may seem old, to others 70 may seem young, and you're both right. Age is relative; it's what you do with those years that count the most. Most of you have testosterone levels that are declining already, regardless of whether you know it or not. Many of you are experiencing some of the signs and symptoms that we have covered including fatigue, depression, erectile dysfunction, and metabolic syndrome. Take a look in the mirror. Has your waist size grown to the point that you can hardly see your shoes? Does the way you look (and the way you feel) accurately reflect the age on your birth certificate? Or do you feel as though you are "much too young to feel this damn old?" If you are one of the thousands of men whose biological age differs significantly from your chronological age, there is no better time than now to change it! So let's get out there and do something! Consider this is a call to action, as no one can be responsible for your health but you. It can seem a bit daunting at first, but just like getting into a cold swimming pool, sometimes you just have to jump right in.

Now that you know the many roles that testosterone plays in the body (both what it is supposed to do and the problems it causes when there is too much or too little), it's time to find out what your hormone levels are doing. Testing your hormone levels should be your first step on the road to wellness. There are several resources listed in the appendix that can help you find a place where you can order your own hormone tests or, of course, your doctor can order them for you. As you gather data about yourself, regardless of who orders the tests, we recommend that you start a medical file and keep copies of all of your lab results there so that you have a place where everything is together. As you get ready to test yourself, keep in mind that reference ranges are provided by the lab to give you an idea of where most people fall. In fact, those ranges are created by testing a large population, finding the median score, and extending the "acceptable" values a certain amount above and below the average. If your lab value is within the "reference range," that doesn't mean that everything is ok. It simply means that you aren't unusually low or high. We are advocating that you **optimize** your hormone levels, which generally means that you want to be doing better than most of the population that was tested.

Remember when you were in school and a 70 was a passing grade, but an 80 or even 90 was better? You may be able to pass through life with mediocre hormone levels, but you don't want to be just getting by, you

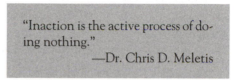

"Inaction is the active process of doing nothing."
                                    —Dr. Chris D. Meletis

want to thrive! It may not have affected your life much if you got a C+ in physics back in high school, but your health is one place where you should be striving for straight As. The way that the reference ranges are calculated makes it like being graded on a curve! Just because everyone else has falling hormones doesn't make it feel any better to you, and certainly doesn't help you out!

The sad reality is that a good number of the men who read this book will put it down and not think of it again until they start to see and feel the effects of their declining hormones. A warning about what can happen won't be enough to motivate some people. And a large number of the guys who wait for signs or symptoms will become interested in the topic again only when they start to experience erectile dysfunction or some other diminishing of their "manhood." Now,

you don't need us to tell you how important sex is, and problems achieving and maintaining an erection can have some very adverse effects on your sex life, but our primary concern when it comes to the signs and symptoms of andropause is metabolic syndrome. This prediabetic and cardiovascular condition can **dramatically shorten your life**, not just your romantic evening. Remember that it is much easier to prevent a problem from happening

If you feel like you are sucking wind to keep up with your friends and co-workers in sports, work, and in life in general, it is time to level the playing field. Remember: test, don't guess. Find out where your hormone levels are and do something about it! Don't wait another couple of years and waste more of your life feeling less than optimal.

than it is to clean up the pieces afterward. There is no reason why you have to let your hormone levels slip below optimal, let alone far lower than those of your peers.

Beyond testosterone, there are a number of factors that play a role in men's health, including estrogen levels as they relate to the prostate. Prostate health is a very important part of men's well-being in general as prostate cancer and benign changes to prostate tissue are so prevalent. Some sources have reported that, by the eighth decade, approximately 80 percent of men will have benign prostatic hyperplasia. The National Cancer Institute estimates that by the age of 75 there will be cancerous changes in the prostate tissue of 50 to 75 percent of men.[1] The initial signs and symptoms of prostate enlargement are urinary urgency, frequency, and/or dribbling stream. Estrogen stimulates the proliferation of prostate tissue, and, as you've learned, estrogen is created from testosterone by the aromatase enzyme that is found primarily in fat tissue. Prostate-related issues are one of the primary reasons why it's important to monitor all of the hormones and not just testosterone.

Stereotypically speaking, women are the talkers and men are the doers. So what can **you do** to keep your hormones balanced and your health optimal?

- Reduce your stress levels: meditate, pray, go to yoga, stop cheering for a losing team or whatever stresses you out and fails to give you positive return—whatever you need to find some quiet time.
- Limit exposure to hormones and hormone disruptors in the environment.
- Keep your body fat percentage low.
- Exercise, both cardiovascular and weight-bearing.
- Test your hormone levels: testosterone, DHEA, estrogen, progesterone, and cortisol.
- Test and monitor your blood sugar levels, blood lipid levels, and cardio-vascular risk factors.
- If your hormones levels are low, consider supplementing with bio-identical hormones to achieve optimal physiologic levels.
- Retest your hormones again a few months after starting a new therapy and yearly after that.
- Limit your alcohol intake and reduce or quit smoking.
- Monitor your diet and limit simple carbohydrates, "bad" fats, and pesticides while ensuring that you are getting enough vegetables (antioxidants), protein, and "good" fats.
- Two rules in food choices are (1) try to eat foods that are as close to their natural state as possible; (2) the more colorful your plate, the better variety of antioxidents and nutrients you are getting.

Well, there you are! We wish that we could make it easier for you. We all want to go to the doctor and let them "fix" us, but unfortunately, that's just not the way it works. Optimal health takes some effort and not just on the part of your care providers—it takes serious effort from you. Shouldn't you be the one who is ultimately responsible for your health, as no one can control your activities or your diet the way you can? Though we do advocate for the use of testosterone (and other hormones such as progesterone) supplementation as necessary for optimum health, we warn that this is not a cure-all. To really "be the best you can be," you'll probably want to employ a combination of these factors. Good luck! You now have the basic knowledge you need. It's up to you to use it.

NOTE

1. National Cancer Institute, *Understanding Prostate Changes: A Health Guide for All Men*, Washington, DC: Public Health Services, 1998; U.S. Dept of Health and Human Services, NIH publication 98-4303.

Resources

LABORATORIES AND TESTING RESOURCES:

www.hischangeoflife.com
This is our site that we created for you to keep up on the latest research and to give you the edge when it comes to devouring life to its fullest. If you are looking for a place to order test results on your own, this is the place to go. As a dynamic educational and empowering resource for men and women, this Web site provides critical and updated life-transforming knowledge, access to and information about a wide variety of tests and supplements, and free discussion forums about the most pressing modern health issues and how to achieve optimal health.

Labrix Clinical Services: www.labrix.com
A laboratory that sets the standard for saliva hormone testing with reliable, fast, and accurate results. In addition to saliva testing, they also offer a 24-hour urine iodine challenge as well as a number of serum hormone tests including a thyroid panel and IGF-1 test. You cannot order the test kits directly from the Web site, but they do have a lot of informative content to help you on your journey.

COMPOUNDING PHARMACIES

Lloyd Center Pharmacy: www.lcrx.com
A full-service compounding pharmacy, their Web site provides information and frequently asked questions about many hormone therapies.

College Pharmacy: www.collegepharmacy.com
For 30 years, this pharmacy has been a leader in compounding individual medications for their patients and their physicians. The Web site is a good general resource on bio-identical hormone therapies.

Medaus Pharmacy: www.medaus.com
A national compounding pharmacy whose Web site includes a physician finder as well as a wealth of information about bio-identical hormone replacement and antiaging therapies.

The International Academy of Compounding Pharmacists (IACP): www.iacprx.org
This organization serves to protect and promote compounding pharmacists and the right for patients to receive individualized prescriptions.

OTHER RESOURCES:

www.DrMeletis.com
Links to a number of national articles, books, and free educational materials designed to provide visitors with quality information regarding optimal health to aid them on their journey to achieve wellness.

www.CPMedical.net
Access Pin# 587556 to get registered. This is a great resource with free articles, quality herbs, lab testing, nutritional products, and health resources.

American College for Advancement in Medicine (ACAM): www.acam.org
"The voice of integrative medicine." This is a good resource to find a doctor who is familiar with bio-identical hormone replacement therapy.

The Institute for Healthy Aging: www.The IHA.org
A nonprofit designed to provide education on natural medicine and be a resource for the media to disseminate information nationally. Interviews for the media can be arranged with physicians on natural medicine health topics.

American Association of Naturopathic Physicians (AANP): www.naturopathic.org
This site can provide you with a general overview of naturopathic medicine as well as guide you in locating an ND near you.

John R. Lee, MD: www.drjohnlee.com
One of the foremost authorities on the uses of progesterone and bio-identical hormone replacement therapy; Dr. Lee's Web site continues his message with a wealth of information for patients and practitioners of all levels.

The Institute for Functional Medicine (IFM): www.functionalmedicine.org
An organization that promotes individualized health care and proactive health, this site is a great resource for finding physicians who share the preventative approach to health.

American Academy of Anti-Aging Medicine (A4M): www.worldhealth.net
A nonprofit organization and community of physicians dedicated to treating the processes of aging.

BOOKS AND RECOMMENDED READING

Slim, Sane & Sexy: Pocket Guide to Natural Bioidentical Hormone Balancing by Jay H. Mead, MD and Erin T. Lommen, ND
A straight talk guide to women's hormones and bio-identical hormone replacement.
Why Zebras Don't Get Ulcers by Robert M. Sapolsky
A comprehensive look at how prolonged stress causes a range of physical and mental conditions.

Hormone Balance Made Simple: The Essential How-to Guide to Symptoms, Dosage, Timing and More by John R. Lee, MD and Virginia Hopkins

Clear and concise guide to hormone balancing for women including quick tests to determine hormone imbalances, details on bio-identical hormones as well as how diet, stress, and lifestyle may affect hormone balance.

Idoine: Why You Need It, Why You Can't Live Without It by David Brownstein, MD

This book provides the much-needed information on the epidemic of iodine deficiency and what that means to your health.

The Abs Diet by David Zinczenko

Much more than a diet book, this is an outline of optimal health with a detailed diet and exercise regimen that is written by the editor in chief of *Men's Health* magazine.

Index

About the Authors

CHRIS D. MELETIS, N.D., is Executive Director of the Institute for Healthy Aging. An internationally recognized educator, author, and lecturer, he also serves as Series Editor for the Praeger series in Complementary and Alternative Medicine. Named the 2003 Naturopathic Physician of the Year by the American Association of Naturopathic Physicians, he is also former Chief Medical Officer and Dean of Naturopathic Medicine at the National College of Naturopathic Medicine. Meletis is Founder of Divine Medicine, an organization dedicated to helping the medically underserved.

SARA G. WOOD, N.D., is a naturopathic physician in private practice in Oregon. Degreed in biochemistry as well as naturopathic medicine, she is also Staff Physician at Labrix Clinical Services, a state-of-the-art laboratory that tests hormone levels in saliva. Her patients include both men and women.